D1242845

URINARY AND FECAL INCONTINENCE

NURSING MANAGEMENT

URINARY AND FECAL INCONTINENCE

NURSING MANAGEMENT

Edited by

DOROTHY B. DOUGHTY, RN, MN, ET

Program Director,
Enterostomal Therapy Nursing Education Program,
Emory University, Atlanta, Georgia

With 88 illustrations

Coordinated with assistance from the
International Association for Enterostomal Therapy

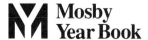

Mosby
Year Book

St. Louis   Baltimore   Boston   Chicago   London   Philadelphia   Sydney   Toronto

618.97
DOU
1991

**Mosby
Year Book**
Dedicated to Publishing Excellence

Editor: Don Ladig, Theresa Van Schaik
Developmental Editor: Jeanne Rowland
Production Manager: Patricia Tannian
Production Editor: Mary McAuley
Book and Cover Design: Gail Morey Hudson

Printed in the United States of America

Mosby−Year Book, Inc.
11830 Westline Industrial Drive, St. Louis, Missouri 63146

Library of Congress Cataloging in Publication Data

Urinary and fecal incontinence: nursing management / [edited by]
   Dorothy B. Doughty; coordinated with assistance from the
International Association for Enterostomal Therapy.
        p.   cm.
    Includes bibliographical references and index.
    ISBN 0-8016-1444-9
    1. Urinary incontinence—Nursing. 2. Fecal incontinence—Nursing.
I. Doughty, Dorothy Beckley. II. International Association for
Enterostomal Therapy.
    [DNLM: 1. Fecal Incontinence—nursing. 2. Urinary Incontinence—
nursing.   WY 164 U76]
RC921.I5U74 1991
618.97'66—dc20
DNLM/DLC
for Library of Congress   91-14156
                                                               CIP

GW/MV 9 8 7 6 5 4 3 2 1

Editorial Board

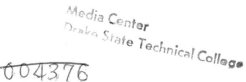

Contributors

ALAN BAKST, Pharm D

Drug Information Specialist,
Pharmacy Educational Services,
Cleveland Clinic Foundation,
Cleveland, Ohio

ALICE BASCH, MSN, RN, ET, OCN

Private Practice,
Santa Rosa, California

JERRY G. BLAIVAS, MD

Professor and Vice-Chairman, Department of Urology,
Director of Neurourology, Squier Urological Clinic,
The Presbyterian Hospital in the City of New York,
New York, New York

NANCY FALLER, BSN, RN, CETN

Enterostomal Therapy Nurse,
Rutland Regional Medical Center, Rutland, Vermont

MIKEL L. GRAY, PhD, CURN

Director, Continence Clinic at Shepherd Spinal Center;
Associate Faculty, Emory Enterostomal Therapy
Nursing Education Program, Emory University,
Atlanta, Georgia

STEPHEN B. HANAUER, MD

Associate Professor of Medicine,
Department of Medicine, Section of Gastroenterology,
University of Chicago, Chicago, Illinois

BARBARA HOCEVAR, BSN, RN, CETN

Enterostomal Therapy Nurse, Cleveland Clinic Foundation,
Cleveland, Ohio

LINDA JENSEN, RN

Clinical Research Director, Colon and Rectal Surgery Associates,
St. Paul, Minnesota

JAMES H. MacLEOD, MD

Attending Surgeon, Intercommunity Presbyterian Hospital,
Whittier, California

LESLIE OLIVER, BS, RN

Urology Nurse Clinician, Squier Urological Clinic,
The Presbyterian Hospital in the City of New York,
New York, New York

MARY JANE PETERS, RN

Urology Nurse Clinician, Loyola University Medical Center,
Maywood, Illinois

DAVID A. ROTHENBERGER, MD

Clinical Professor of Surgery, Division of Colon and Rectal Surgery,
University of Minnesota, Minneapolis, Minnesota

KAREN S. SABLE, MD

Fellow, Gastroenterology, University of Chicago Medical Center,
Chicago, Illinois

ELLEN SHIPES, MN, MEd, RN, CETN

Enterostomal Therapy Nurse, Veterans Administration Medical Center,
Nashville, Tennessee

STEVEN SIEGEL, MD

Department of Urology, Cleveland Clinic Foundation,
Cleveland, Ohio

RICHARD TROY, MD

Department of Urology, Cleveland Clinic Foundation,
Cleveland, Ohio

JOHN S. WHEELER, Jr., MD

Associate Professor of Urology, Loyola University Medical Center,
Maywood, Illinois

Preface

Incontinence is gaining recognition as a major health care problem. It is difficult to accurately determine the number of persons who have incontinence, because many have had no evaluation or treatment; however, the National Institutes of Health estimate that at least 10 million adult Americans are incontinent.* Urinary incontinence appears to be epidemic among the elderly: approximately half of the residents in nursing homes and 15% to 30% of elderly persons living in the community are incontinent.* Even less data are available regarding the number of persons with fecal incontinence.

Although determining the *quantitative* impact of incontinence is difficult, patients have clearly described the *qualitative* impact. In a society that emphasizes continence and cleanliness, where elimination processes are joked about but rarely discussed openly, incontinence restricts the life-style of patients and imposes psychologic pain. Patients report feelings of embarrassment, shame, isolation, helplessness, and loss of self-esteem. Incontinence affects every aspect of daily life: clothing selection, decisions about food and fluid intake, occupational choices, leisure activities and travel, and sexual activities and intimacy. The difficulties encountered in living with incontinence also affect the patients' families; family members share the pain, frustration, and limitations. In addition, the management of incontinence can create a financial burden; an estimated 10 billion dollars is spent annually on the management of urinary incontinence alone.*

Until recently, one of the biggest obstacles to the effective management of incontinence has been the perception that incontinence was inevitable and

---

*National Institutes of Health: *Consensus Conference on Urinary Incontinence in Adults,* Kansas City, Mo, 1989, Marion Laboratories.

irreversible, a perception almost as common among health care providers as patients. Thus "management" usually meant containment and odor control and was more likely to be handled with mail-order supplies than with the help of the health care professional.

We now know that incontinence is a *symptom* and that with accurate diagnosis and appropriate management most cases of incontinence can be reversed or effectively managed. We also now recognize that, although changes associated with aging make the older person more susceptible to incontinence, loss of continence is *not* a normal part of the aging process. Incontinence in an older person should always be assessed carefully so that appropriate treatment can be initiated.

A multidisciplinary focus is necessary in incontinence management so that each patient is offered comprehensive evaluation, accurate diagnosis, and appropriate treatment. Nurses have much to offer these patients; by virtue of our role in patient care, we are often the first to detect a problem with bowel or bladder function, and our holistic focus facilitates the assessment, teaching, and support that are critical to the diagnosis and management of the problem. Nurses can offer much more than sympathy, containment, and skin protection: we can contribute significantly to detection, assessment, and management. To do so, we must acquire a strong knowledge base that incorporates an understanding of normal physiology, common pathophysiologic mechanisms, and available treatments. This text is designed to broaden the nurse's knowledge base in each of these areas.

Written by ET nurses and other incontinence specialists, this text is divided into two sections: management of urinary incontinence and management of fecal incontinence. Each section begins with a review of normal physiology and then describes common pathophysiologic processes; subsequent chapters on assessment and management are based on the preceding discussion of normal physiology and potential alterations. Each chapter concludes with a self-evaluation, which can be used in two ways: (1) The reader may choose to use the self-evaluation as a pretest. If he or she is able to answer most of the questions correctly, further study of the chapter may not be necessary. (2) The reader may conclude a study of the chapter by using the self-evaluation as a posttest, to assess his or her mastery of the content.

Acknowledgments

I extend sincere appreciation to the following people; without their help this book would not have been possible:

My husband and sons, who kept the word processor working, stepped over the paper stacks, and accepted my frequent nonavailability

The editorial board, for their marathon weekend work: Donna Brewer, Ruth Bryant, Beverly Hampton, Michiko Ooka, and Joan Van Niel (special thanks to Ruth Bryant for editorial support and assistance)

Jeanne Rowland, nursing developmental editor, for her untiring patience, consistent availability, sense of humor, and invaluable assistance

The people at Convatec, for their generous financial support of the project

Dorothy B. Doughty

Contents

URINARY AND FECAL INCONTINENCE

NURSING MANAGEMENT

1 Anatomy and Physiology of Voiding

JOHN S. WHEELER, JR.
MARY JANE PETERS

OBJECTIVES

1. Identify the structures that secure and support the bladder and bladder neck in the correct anatomic position.
2. Explain the importance of normal support for the bladder neck.
3. Explain the significance of normal bladder wall compliance.
4. Differentiate the internal from the external sphincter mechanism by location and type of musculature and control.
5. Identify factors that support continence in the female.
6. Explain the role of the prostate gland in maintaining continence and in dysfunctional voiding.
7. Explain the role of the parasympathetic, sympathetic, and somatic nerves in mediating normal bladder storage and emptying.
8. Trace the pathways for parasympathetic, sympathetic, and somatic innervation, and explain how neurologic lesions affect bladder function.
9. Describe the normal micturition reflex.
10. Describe age-related changes in bladder function, including the following:
    Neonatal bladder function and the acquisition of continence
    Effects of puberty
    Effects of prostate hyperplasia in the male and menopause in the female.

Knowledge of the anatomy and physiology of the normal lower urinary tract is the key to understanding the causes, diagnosis, and management of urinary incontinence. Currently, most techniques of management are intended to re-establish the normal function of the lower urinary tract. The lower urinary tract consists of the bladder and urethra, which are confined and well supported within the pelvis. The lower urinary tract is controlled by the central nervous system through the parasympathetic, sympathetic, and somatic nerve pathways. Normal function of the lower urinary tract requires a complex integration of all nerve pathways and enables the person to store and empty urine normally.

ANATOMY OF LOWER URINARY TRACT
Bladder and Support Structures

The urinary bladder is extraperitoneal and lies at the base of the pelvis on the pelvic floor. The bladder neck in men is secured by its adherence to the endopelvic fascia and the prostate gland; in women, support for the bladder neck is provided by the endopelvic fascia and its connections to the pelvic floor, urethra, rectum, and vagina (Figs. 1-1 and 1-2). The ureters, vesical arteries, obliterated umbilical artery, and peritoneal reflection over the bladder dome also secure the position of the bladder. In men the peritoneal connection to the bladder is freely distensible; in women it is indented by the uterus.

Pelvic Floor Muscles and Ligaments

The muscles of the pelvic floor include the levator ani, coccygeus, internal obturator, pyriform, and superficial and deep perineal muscles, which are also known as the urogenital diaphragm (Fig. 1-3). These muscles are attached to the pubic bone and ischium; they encircle and help support the urethra, vagina, and rectum. Voluntary contraction of these muscles results in compression, lengthening, and elevation of the urethra. For example, voiding can be interrupted by contracting the pubococcygeal muscle. The deep perineal muscles of the urogenital diaphragm are attached to the pubic arch superiorly and surround the membranous urethra as the external skeletal muscle sphincter, a structure important to continence.

Anterior to the bladder is the prevesical retropubic space of Retzius, which contains fatty tissue and important blood vessels that lead to the bladder, prostate, and genitalia. The space of Retzius allows easy surgical access to the bladder and prostate. (This space is the area of exposure for the Marshall-Marchetti-Krantz procedure, a method of urethropexy that corrects urinary stress incontinence in women.) At the inferolateral borders of this space are the puboprostatic ligaments (in men) and the pubourethral ligaments (in women);

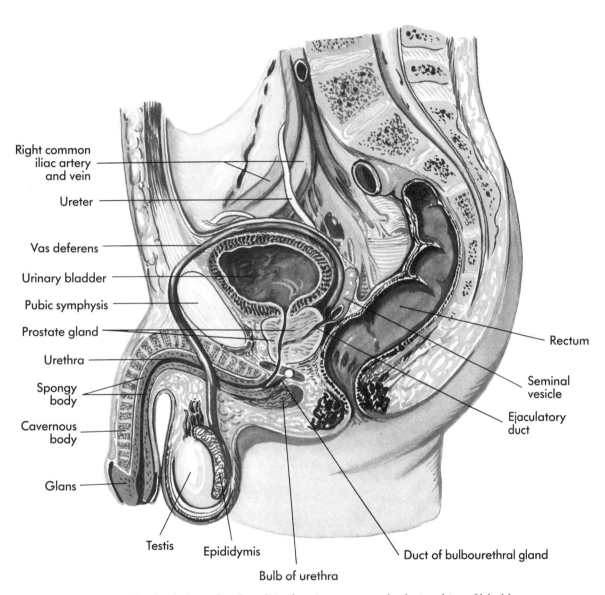

Fig. 1-1   Sagittal view of male pelvis showing structural relationships of bladder, urethra, and prostate gland with some of their attachments to pelvic floor. (From Anthony C and Thibodeau G: Textbook of anatomy and physiology, ed 12, St Louis, 1987, Mosby–Year Book, Inc.)

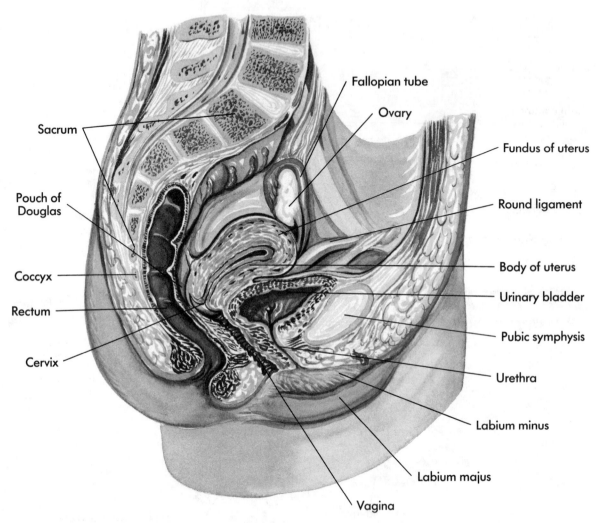

Fig. 1-2   Sagittal view of female pelvis showing structural relationships of bladder, urethra, and vagina with some of their attachments to pelvic floor. (From Anthony C and Thibodeau G: Textbook of anatomy and physiology, ed 12, St Louis, 1987, Mosby–Year Book, Inc.)

these ligaments represent thickenings of the endopelvic fascia that covers the levators. These ligaments secure the anterior lower urinary tract to the pubic bone and are important surgical landmarks.

The bladder's posterolateral surface lies on the levator ani and obturator internus muscles. This surface is anterior to the rectum and is separated from the rectum in the male by the vas deferens, seminal vesicles, and prostate, all of which are surrounded by Denonvilliers' fascia, the rectovesical fascia (Fig. 1-1). During a prostatectomy, Denonvilliers' fascia is an important surgical landmark.

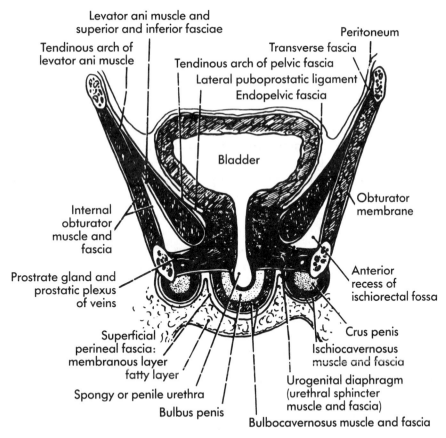

Fig. 1-3   Frontal section of male pelvis showing pelvic floor muscles and external sphincter and their relationships to urinary tract. (From Boyarsky S: Neurogenic bladder, Baltimore, 1967, Williams & Wilkins.)

Prostate Gland and Urethra of Male

In men the prostate gland is important in maintaining continence; it is also frequently involved in diseases and disorders (Figs. 1-1 and 1-3). The prostate gland, a firm, fibromuscular capsular structure, is normally the size of a chestnut. Its interior is glandular, and the gland hypertrophies with age. The urethra traverses the prostate, exits at the prostate apex, and continues into the membranous urethra, which joins the rest of the perineal urethra. Into the distal prostatic urethra projects the verumontanum, which contains the openings of the ejaculatory duct and serves as a landmark during transurethral prostate surgery. Because the verumontanum is adjacent to the external sphincter, inadvertent resection distal to the verumontanum may result in postoperative incontinence.

The prostatic urethra contains both smooth and striated muscle. The smooth muscle comes from the bladder trigone and extends down through the proximal urethra into the prostate.[4] The striated muscle is an extension of the deep perineal muscles (the urogenital diaphragm) and extends into the apex of the prostate. This striated muscle is known as the rhabdosphincter, which in conjunction with the urogenital diaphragm is the external sphincter mechanism. Its specific role in the maintenance of continence is controversial and still under investigation.[*]

The urethra in the male has several distinct anatomic sections: the prostatic urethra, membranous urethra, bulbous urethra, and pendulous urethra. As previously stated, the prostatic urethra is the portion that traverses the prostate gland and continues into the membranous urethra. The membranous urethra, approximately 1.5 to 2.0 cm in length, is the most fixed part of the urethra: it is firmly attached to the urogenital diaphragm. Because the membranous urethra is so firmly attached, it is the part of the urethra most susceptible to injury with pelvic trauma. The membranous urethra continues into the anterior urethra, which includes the bulbous urethra of the perineum, pendulous urethra (penile urethra), navicular fossa (urethra within the glans penis), and urethral meatus (Figs. 1-1 and 1-3). The bulbocavernosus and ischiocavernosus skeletal muscles in the superficial perineal area and the rectourethral muscle in the deep perineum provide indirect urethral resistance at the level of the membranous and bulbous urethra.

Bladder Neck and Urethra of Female

In women the bladder neck is attached to the inferior pubis by the pubourethral ligaments. These ligaments, which stabilize the proximal urethra, help preserve the integrity of the bladder neck and maintain continence. Other pelvic ligaments that support the uterus and vagina include the pubocervical liga-

---

*References, 5, 8, 11, 18, 20, and 22.

ments, which extend from the cervix to the pubis; the lateral cervical ligaments and broad ligaments, which extend from the lateral cervix and upper vagina to the pelvic sidewalls; the uteral sacral ligaments, which extend from the back of the uterus to the sacrum; and the uterine (round) ligaments, which attach the uterine wall to the inguinal area (Fig. 1-2). Defects in any one of these structures can lead to incontinence. For example, a herniation of the bladder or urethra through the pubocervical fascia, by definition a cystocele or urethrocele, appears as a protrusion of the bladder or urethra into the vagina and may be associated with incontinence caused by loss of structural integrity.

The urethra of the female is not as complex as that of the male for two reasons: in women the two sphincters are not well defined and they are deficient in muscle thickness posteriorly (Fig. 1-4). Therefore urethral resistance depends more on the normally competent bladder neck and proximal urethra (the internal sphincter) and less on the poorly developed external sphincter. The muscles of the pelvic floor in women, modulated by the ovarian hormone, estrogen, indirectly promote continence. In premenopausal women, estrogen helps maintain the tone of these structures by stimulating the estrogen receptors in the

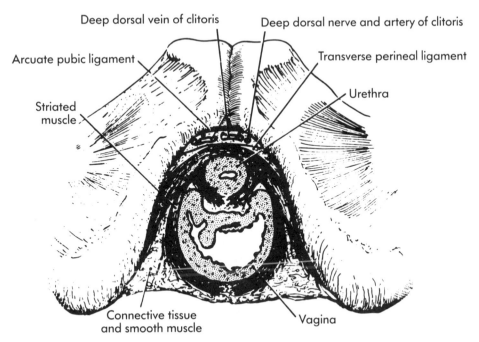

Fig. 1-4 Cross section of female pelvis showing relationships of urethra and vagina to the pelvic floor and deficient posterior external sphincter. (From Boyarsky S: Neurogenic bladder, Baltimore, 1967, Williams & Wilkins.)

pelvic floor and urethra.[3,19] The distal urethra of the female is less than 2 cm in length (total length of the urethra, 4 cm) and contributes little support to continence. The structure of the urethral wall, however, does provide support that helps maintain continence. The softness of the inner urethral wall allows it to mold and form a watertight seal in the resting state and promotes coaptation of the urethral mucosa.[9] The urethral wall also provides tension that compresses these coapting mucosal walls.[23] These functions depend on the structural integrity of the urethral wall, which includes fibroelastic tissue and the striated and smooth muscle around the urethral mucosa.[23] Because of these urethral properties, passive tonic urethral resistance is normally well maintained.

Other anatomic features that help promote continence in women are (1) a normal angle from the urethra to the bladder neck (urethrovesical angle), (2) a normal vertical urethral angle, and (3) normal urethral length. The normal urethrovesical angle is 90 degrees; the normal vertical urethral angle is 30 degrees. The presence of these normal angles indicates a well-supported bladder and urethra. Increases in the vertical urethral angle (to more than 30 degrees) may indicate loss of urethral support with increased urethral mobility. Increases in the urethrovesical angle (to more than 100 degrees) may indicate poor funneling of the bladder neck. These two abnormalities suggest poor pelvic support and may be associated with incontinence. As stated previously, the urethra is normally more than 4 cm long, but the functional length, that is, the length of the urethra that helps maintain resistance and prevent incontinence, is usually about 2 cm.

Bladder Muscle

The full bladder is a spherical structure composed of trigonal smooth muscle superimposed upon three layers of intertwining smooth muscle (Fig. 1-5). The bladder is normally a compliant structure that allows adequate filling (up to an average of 400 ml) and complete emptying. Factors that reduce compliance include the thickening of the bladder wall and the increase in fibrous tissue caused by overactivity of the bladder and high intravesical pressure, and chronic inflammation, which thickens the mucosa of the bladder.

The trigone muscle is the most fixed aspect of the bladder base. The lateral wings of the trigone are the entrance points of the two ureters, which course to the bladder through narrow tunnels (1 cm in width) in the bladder wall and end at the trigone. This anatomic relationship normally prevents ureteral reflux. The trigone is far more prominent in men than in women. The trigone musculature continues into the circumferential smooth muscle of the proximal urethra.[4] The trigone and bladder neck function as the bladder base, and the rest of the bladder, including the dome, is known as the bladder body.[8,9] The interior of the bladder is covered by loose, transitional cell surface mucosa

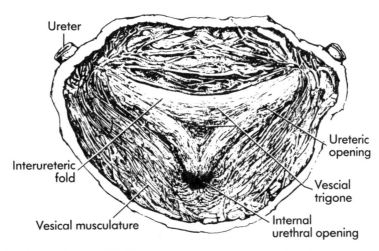

Ureter

Ureteric opening

Interureteric fold

Vescial trigone

Vesical musculature

Internal urethral opening

Fig. 1-5 Open view of bladder showing trigone and related structures. (From Boyarsky S: Neurogenic bladder, Baltimore, 1967, Williams & Wilkins.)

similar to the mucosa in the proximal urethra; the mucosa attaches to the submucosa, which is attached to the muscle wall.

As mentioned previously, the proximal urethra has two sphincters that differ in function. The internal sphincter mechanism at the bladder neck is the smooth-muscle sphincter, whereas the external sphincter mechanism is made up of striated skeletal muscle (the urogenital diaphragm).

NEUROLOGIC CONTROL OF LOWER URINARY TRACT

The nerve supply to the lower urinary tract includes parasympathetic, sympathetic, and somatic nerve fibers (Fig. 1-6). Neurotransmitters released at the neuromuscular junctions are received by neuroreceptors located throughout the lower urinary tract (Table 1-1). Neurotransmitters and neuropeptides that have been identified and may prove to be important in altering urinary tract function include prostaglandins, purine nucleotides such as adenosine triphosphate (ATP), histamine, serotonin, vasoactive intestinal peptides, enkephalins, and substance P and other tachykinins.[5,7,13]

Parasympathetic Innervation

The parasympathetic system provides motor stimulation to the bladder and mediates bladder contraction via the pelvic nerve. The pelvic nerve exits the spinal cord at the level of the sacral cord (S2-4), the conus medullaris. (The

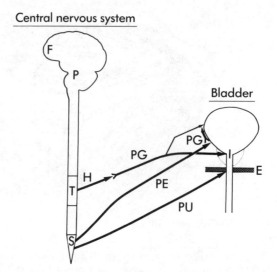

Fig. 1-6   Schema of neuroanatomy of lower urinary tract. *F*, Frontal cortex; *P*, pons; *T*, thoracic spinal cord; *S*, sacral spinal cord; *H*, hypogastric nerve; *PE*, pelvic nerve; *PU*, pudendal nerve; *E*, external sphincter; *I*, internal sphincter; *PG*, post-ganglionic nerve. Prostate gland is outlined in dots. (From Wheeler JS, Niecestro RM, and Goggin C: J Enterost Ther 15[6]:241, 1988.)

sacral cord level is actually the thoracic-lumbar [T12-L1] vertebral body level.) The preganglionic nerve originates in the nucleus of the sacral detrusor in the intermediolateral region of the sacral cord and courses along the rectum to the bladder base; the short postganglionic nerve is within the bladder wall.

Sympathetic Innervation

The sympathetic nerves originate in the thoracic and lumbar cord (T11-L2), course along the great vessels, and synapse at the inferior mesenteric and hypogastric plexuses. The postganglionic hypogastric nerve travels to the bladder neck and proximal urethra, the primary sites for sympathetic stimulation. Some of these fibers also innervate the body of the bladder and indirectly affect the parasympathetic nerves. The sympathetic nerves mediate bladder storage, primarily by stimulating contractions in the bladder neck and proximal urethra.

Somatic Innervation

Efferent (Motor) Innervation. Efferent fibers of the somatic nervous system originate from the pudendal nucleus (S2-4) in the ventral horn of the sacral cord and course along the autonomic nerves to innervate the external striated

Table 1-1   Neurotransmitters that mediate micturition

Neurotransmitter	Innervation	Neuroreceptor	Location of neuroreceptor	Physiologic effect
Acetylcholine	Somatic	Cholinergic	External sphincter	Bladder storage
Acetylcholine	Parasympathetic	Cholinergic	Bladder base and body	Bladder contraction
Norepinephrine	Sympathetic	Adrenergic	Alpha: bladder base, neck, and proximal urethra	Bladder storage
			Beta: bladder body	Bladder storage

muscle sphincter and the muscles of the pelvic floor. These efferent fibers support bladder storage by effecting contraction of the external sphincter.

Afferent (Sensory) Innervation. Afferent innervation proceeds from the bladder through the pelvic and hypogastric nerves into the dorsal horn of the spinal cord; it continues into complex local, sacral connections (to initiate local reflexes) or to the brain via the spinothalamic tract. These pathways transmit impulses that produce sensation and permit voluntary control of the bladder.[13] Sensory fibers along the pelvic nerve are stimulated during filling via mechanoreceptors in the bladder muscle. Sensory fibers along the hypogastric and pudendal nerves transmit impulses that produce sensations of pain and regulate temperature in the bladder's mucosa.[5]

Neural Coordination of Micturition

The central nervous system controls normal micturition. Originally it was thought that the spinal cord operated independently and could coordinate detrusor and sphincter activity. Although a reflex contraction of the bladder can be generated from the sacral cord, we now know that the cord alone cannot coordinate the complex process of micturition.[1,2,6,12]

Normal Micturition Reflex. During the micturition reflex, sensory stimulation passes from the bladder into and through the sacral cord and is coordinated in the rostral pontine reticular formation of the brain, that is, the pons. The pons coordinates the relaxation of the urethral sphincter just before a normal detrusor contraction.[1,2,6,12] The pons is controlled voluntarily by the frontal cortex, which can either facilitate or inhibit pontine activity. Hence, voluntary control of the detrusor is transmitted from the frontal cortex through the pons down the reticulospinal tract to the detrusor nucleus and effectively inhibits the detrusor. Without this cerebrocortical control the bladder's activity would be involuntary and uninhibited, like the bladder activity of an infant with undeveloped cerebral control of bladder function. Direct corticospinal connections from the frontal cortex to the pudendal nucleus in the sacral cord also provide voluntary control of the external sphincter.

Effect of Neurologic Lesions on Micturition. Knowing that the pons coordinates the function of the bladder and the urethral sphincters, the nurse can understand the patterns of bladder function associated with certain neurologic lesions. For example, a patient with a stroke located in the frontal cerebral cortex has a loss of cortical inhibition to the pons that results in uninhibited detrusor activity, that is, detrusor hyperreflexia. However, coordination between the bladder and the sphincters continues in such a patient because the pontine sacral axis has been preserved. This pattern of detrusor hyperreflexia causes the symptoms of frequency, urgency, and incontinence that are seen in patients with neurologic lesions such as stroke. A lesion below the pontine level (for example, a spinal cord injury) results in a loss of coordinated bladder-sphincter activity (bladder-sphincter dyssynergia), because the pontine sacral axis has been disrupted. This common finding in patients with spinal cord injury, if not treated, can lead to such diseases of the upper urinary tract as pyelonephritis, hydronephrosis, stone disease, and renal insufficiency.

NORMAL MICTURITION

The normal micturition reflex includes a phase of filling and storage and a phase of contraction and emptying.

Filling Phase

During the filling phase, bladder pressure rises slowly, depending on normal compliance of the bladder wall, and there is little cholinergic activity. The normal integrity of the pelvic floor and the urethra provides passive urethral resistance to help maintain continence; this resistance is amplified by tonic sympathetic activity. At a critical bladder pressure and volume (usually 300 to 400 ml), the person feels an urge to void; this urge represents the micturition threshold. At this point, sympathetic stimulation increases, resulting in (1) contraction of the internal sphincter via alpha-adrenergic reception, which increases urethral resistance, and (2) suppression of bladder activity via beta-adrenergic reception, which inhibits bladder contractility. The increased sympathetic stimulation promotes continence. Pudendal nerve activity also increases, resulting in the voluntary contraction of the external urethral sphincter known as the guarding reflex, which further increases urethral resistance and promotes continence.[17] This sequence of events depends on low intravesical pressure, normal bladder sensation, and absence of involuntary bladder activity.

Emptying Phase

Eventually, bladder distention causes increased sensory afferent stimulation, which leads to coordinated micturition. Voluntary inhibition of the somatic discharge to the striated external sphincter decreases resistance at the urinary outlet. Sympathetic nerve activity decreases, causing relaxation of the bladder neck and proximal urethra and unopposed facilitation of parasympathetic stimulation. Parasympathetic stimulation further opens the bladder neck and promotes bladder contraction. With increased bladder pressure and decreased urethral resistance, normal voiding ensues.

This coordinated micturition reflex is controlled by the pons and modulated by the frontal cerebral cortex to provide voluntary micturition. A normal voiding pattern includes decreased urethral sphincter resistance, absence of urinary outlet obstruction, and minimal residual urine (less than 20 ml). Interference with this normal pattern anywhere from the central nervous system to the bladder wall and urethra can cause voiding dysfunction.

Normal Cystometry and Electromyography

The normal voiding pattern can be recorded easily by basic simultaneous cystometry and electromyography (Fig. 1-7). The cystometrogram (CMG) mea-

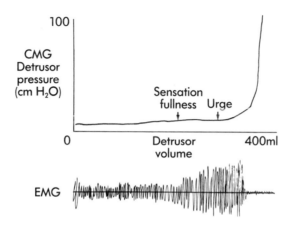

Fig. 1-7 Normal results of CMG and EMG. (From Wheeler JS, Niecestro RM, and Goggin C: J Enterost Ther 15[6]:244, 1988.)

sures bladder function and the electromyogram (EMG) records the activity of muscle in the pelvic floor and sphincter. The normal voiding pattern recorded by the CMG shows a low bladder pressure at low bladder volumes; as the bladder fills to a volume of 300 to 400 ml, the patient feels a sensation of fullness and then urgency. The EMG is nonspecific; it reveals increasing muscle activity in the pelvic floor when the patient first feels the urge to void. This increasing activity in the pelvic floor is the guarding reflex discussed earlier.[17] At the micturition threshold the EMG is silent and the CMG shows a rapid change in bladder pressure, which indicates a bladder contraction with appropriate sphincter relaxation. This is the normal, voluntary voiding pattern, as measured by the CMG and EMG.

AGE-RELATED FACTORS IN VOIDING
Normal Development In Utero

The bladder and urethra develop from the anterior cloaca, or the urogenital sinus; the superior aspect becomes the bladder, and the inferior aspect becomes the urethra. The posterior urethra (prostate and membranous urethra) in the male at the embryonic stage is similar to the entire urethra of the female at the same stage. Normal sexual development in utero results in the gender-specific characteristics of the lower urinary tracts of the male and female.

Neonatal Bladder Function

The neonate normally voids within the first 24 hours after birth. The specific neuropharmacologic activity of the neonatal bladder is not well understood, but neurotransmitters are sparse.[10] This sparsity and the immaturity of the central nervous system cause the typical pattern of uninhibited contraction of the detrusor in the neonatal bladder.[10] The bladder accommodates minimal filling and then is emptied by coordinated micturition with little voluntary control.

Acquisition of Continence

Between the ages of 2 and 3, as the child's neuromuscular and mental capabilities mature, greater facilitory and inhibitory control of the bladder, urethra, and pelvic floor develops. Most children are trained by the age of 3 to control the bladder and use the toilet during the day. However, it is common for children up to 4 and 5 years of age to have "accidents" during the day and nocturnal enuresis; this information alleviates the concerns of many parents.

Puberty

The genitalia do not mature in boys and girls until puberty, when the pelvic genitalia also become functional. The prostate gland in an infant boy is small, but the gland grows large enough by puberty to assist with ejaculation. With growth, the prostate gland provides further support for the pelvic floor and urethral resistance. When a girl reaches puberty, the structures of her pelvic floor mature. With estrogenic influence, estrogen receptors of the urethra and pelvic floor in women help maintain pelvic floor tone and increase urethral resistance.[3,19]

Adult Male

Prostate Growth. Until the age of 40, the prostate gland grows slowly and few voiding problems occur. After the age of 40 to 45, into the seventh, eighth, or even ninth decade, the growth of the prostate gland accelerates. The cause of this growth spurt is not well understood, but the growth is presumably due to a change in the balance of hormones in aging men that alters the hormonal milieu of the prostate gland.

Impact of Prostate Hypertrophy. With prostate enlargement the base of the bladder can become distorted, and obstructing tissue can cause increasing urethral resistance. Voiding patterns vary, depending on the severity of the obstruction. The increased contractility required to effect voiding through the highly resistant system causes the bladder to become hypertrophied relatively quickly. The patient exhibits prostatism, a condition marked by symptoms of frequency, urgency, and nocturia. If the obstruction continues, the bladder can decompensate and urinary retention may develop.

Factors that Affect Continence. The patient with prostate enlargement may exhibit involuntary bladder activity that causes urge incontinence, and overflow (paradoxical) incontinence may later develop. Usually, surgical correction, that is, a transurethral prostatectomy, is necessary to restore continence and eliminate the urethral obstruction. The voiding abnormalities caused by prostate obstruction can be further complicated late in life by mental deterioration, which may alter the neurotransmission to the urinary tract.[14-16] This alteration can lead to uninhibited bladder activity and cause incontinence.[15,16]

Adult Female

Childbearing Years. Childbirth, especially repeated deliveries, can either temporarily or permanently distort or traumatize the pelvic floor and urethral anatomy in women. If pregnancy and delivery are normal, exercise and the influence of estrogen can usually restore the tone of the pelvic floor and the integrity of the lower urinary tract. However, the pelvic ligaments, muscles, and urethra are stretched during pregnancy and become lax with time, especially after menopause.

Postmenopausal Changes. After menopause, levels of estrogen in the body decrease, causing the structures of the pelvic floor to atrophy and the urethral mucosa to become thin and friable. Reduced support for the pelvic floor may permit herniation of the urinary tract through the paracervical fascia and result in decreased urethral resistance.[14] Decreasing urethral tone and mucosal coaptation further diminish urethral resistance,[14] and significant changes can lead to urinary stress incontinence. In addition, the altered urethral mucosa is more susceptible to infection.[14]

Factors that Affect Continence. Many postmenopausal women have voiding abnormalities; if the abnormalities are severe, they can cause incontinence. Incontinence is especially likely when bladder pressure is increased, for example, during coughing and sneezing. Postmenopausal changes may be accentuated in elderly women with altered cerebrocortical function, resulting in both reduced capacity and uninhibited activity of the bladder.[15,16] Although urinary incontinence is not considered part of the normal aging process and should not be accepted as such, age-related changes are predisposing factors and do make incontinence more likely in older patients.

SUMMARY

Clearly, urinary continence depends on many complex, interacting factors integrated in a well-ordered system. As discussed in this chapter, all the following anatomic and physiologic factors are important:

1. The cerebral cortex, the pons and its connections, and the nuclei and tracts of the spinal cord must be intact.
2. The sympathetic, parasympathetic, and somatic nerve pathways to the lower urinary tract must be intact.
3. The neurotransmitters (adrenergic, cholinergic, and those still being investigated) must be active.
4. The afferent sensory system must be intact to allow normal filling and must not be overly sensitive.
5. The bladder must have a compliant wall to allow filling at low pressure with no uninhibited contractions.
6. The urinary outlet must provide appropriate resistance with no obstruction. Resistance depends on (a) the normal length of the urethra; (b) the normal caliber of the urethra; (c) the natural tension of the urethral wall; (d) the normally supple urethral mucosa (in women, partially estrogen-dependent); and (e) appropriate tonic neurotransmission from the central nervous system.[21] The outlet must be supported by the normally functioning structures of the pelvic floor (ligaments, fascia, and muscles).

All these properties of the urinary tract contribute to normal voiding and continence. An understanding of them determines treatment for patients with incontinence.

SELF-EVALUATION

QUESTIONS

1. Structures that provide support for the bladder and urethra include:
   a. Pelvic floor muscles and pelvic ligaments
   b. Internal and external sphincters
   c. Other pelvic organs and abdominal muscles
   d. Detrusor muscle and pelvic connective tissue
2. Identify the various sections of the urethra in men by anatomic location.
3. Identify at least two factors that contribute to urethral competence in women.
4. a. Define the term "bladder wall compliance."
   b. Explain the significance of normal compliance.
5. Explain the mechanism that prevents vesicoureteral reflex.
6. The bladder muscle (detrusor) is made up of:
   a. Smooth muscle fibers
   b. Striated muscle fibers
   c. A combination of smooth and striated muscle fibers
7. Distinguish between the internal and external sphincter by location, musculature, and neural regulation.
8. Describe the role of the autonomic and somatic nerve pathways in mediating normal bladder function.
9. Trace the neural pathways for autonomic and somatic nerves that affect bladder and sphincter function.
10. Voiding is normally controlled by:
    a. The central nervous system (cerebral cortex)
    b. The spinal cord micturition center
    c. Local bladder and sphincter reflex arcs
11. The pons is responsible for:
    a. Coordinating the relaxation of the urethral sphincter and the contraction of the detrusor
    b. Inhibiting detrusor contractility
    c. Generating reflex bladder contractions
    d. Maintaining closure of the urethral sphincter
12. Explain the effects of the following lesions on voiding:
    a. Cerebrocortical lesion (for example, stroke)
    b. Lesion below the pons (for example, suprasacral spinal cord injury)
13. Identify the two phases of normal micturition.
14. Define the following terms and explain their significance:
    a. Micturition threshold
    b. Guarding reflex
15. Identify the usual sequence of events in coordinated micturition.

16. Explain the neurologic changes that facilitate toilet training.
17. Describe the impact of estrogen on urethral continence in women.
18. Explain the effects of the prostate gland on male continence and describe the gland's role in dysfunctional voiding.
19. Explain why older adults may be more prone to incontinence.

SELF-EVALUATION

ANSWERS

1. **a.** Pelvic floor muscles and pelvic ligaments
2. **a.** Prostatic urethra: the portion of the urethra traversing the prostate gland
   b. Membranous urethra: the portion of the urethra between the prostatic urethra and the bulbous urethra
   c. Bulbous urethra: the perineal portion of the urethra
   d. Pendulous urethra: the portion of the urethra traversing the penile shaft
   e. Navicular fossa: the portion of the urethra within the glans penis
3. **a.** The softness of the inner urethral wall, which causes mucosal coaptation
   b. The urethral musculature
   c. The normal angle of the bladder neck and the urethra (which depends on normal support for its anatomic position) and normal function of the internal sphincter
   d. The normal length of the urethra
   e. The pelvic floor muscles
4. **a.** The ability of the bladder to stretch and store urine while maintaining low intravesical pressure.
   b. Normal compliance supports the filling stage of bladder function. Decreased compliance results in increased bladder pressures and decreased bladder capacity and is associated with incontinence and upper tract damage.
5. The ureters normally enter the bladder through a narrow tunnel (1 cm in width) in the bladder wall.
6. **a.** Smooth muscle fibers
7. **a.** Internal sphincter: the proximal component of the urethral sphincter; located at the bladder neck; made up of smooth muscle; controlled by the autonomic nervous system (sympathetic stimulation increases the tone of the bladder neck and the proximal urethra)
   b. External sphincter: the distal component of the urethral sphincter mechanism; located in the distal prostatic urethra (male) or the proximal urethra (female); composed of striated muscle (a component of the deep perineal muscles known as the urogenital diaphragm); controlled by the somatic nervous system (voluntary control)
8. **a.** **Autonomic-sympathetic nerve pathways** support urine storage by stimulating the bladder neck and proximal urethra.
   b. **Autonomic-parasympathetic nerve pathways** support emptying by stimulating the contraction of the bladder.

    c. **Somatic-afferent nerve pathways** mediate the stretching of the bladder wall and mucosal pain and temperature; provide conscious sensation of the bladder and voluntary bladder control.

    d. **Somatic-efferent nerve pathways** support bladder storage by stimulating the contraction of the external sphincter.

9. a. **Autonomic-sympathetic nerve pathways** originate at the thoracic-lumbar cord (T11-L2); synapse at the inferior mesenteric and hypogastric plexuses; the postganglionic nerve travels to the bladder neck and the proximal urethra. (Some fibers innervate the body of the bladder and indirectly affect parasympathetic nerves.)

    b. **Autonomic-parasympathetic nerve pathways** originate at the sacral cord (S2-4); course along the rectum to the base of the bladder; the postganglionic nerve is located within the bladder wall.

    c. **Somatic-afferent nerve pathways** originate within the bladder wall; course along the autonomic nerves to the spinal cord; set off local reflexes or travel to the brain via the spinothalamic tracts.

    d. **Somatic-efferent nerve pathways** are controlled by the central nervous system (the frontal cortex, via the corticospinal tracts); local fibers originate at the sacral cord (S2-4), that is, the pudendal nucleus in the sacral cord; travel along the autonomic nerves to the muscles of the pelvic floor and the striated (external) sphincter.

10. a. The central nervous system (cerebral cortex)

11. a. Coordinating the relaxation of the urethral sphincter and the contraction of the detrusor

12. a. **Cerebrocortical lesion** (for example, stroke): loss of cortical inhibition, with resultant detrusor hyperreflexia. Bladder-sphincter coordination is unaffected.

    b. **Lesion below the pons** (for example, suprasacral spinal cord injury): loss of bladder-sphincter coordination (that is, bladder-sphincter dyssynergia).

13. a. Bladder filling and storage

    b. Bladder contraction and emptying

14. a. **Micturition threshold:** point during bladder filling at which a person feels the urge to void (in adults the threshold usually occurs at a volume of 300 to 400 ml). At this point, sympathetic stimulation increases and continence is maintained (by the contraction of the internal sphincter and the suppression of bladder contractility).

    b. **Guarding reflex:** the increase in the activity of the pudendal nerve that results in voluntary contraction of the external sphincter; occurs in response to bladder filling.

15. 1. Voluntary inhibition or relaxation of the external sphincter
2. Decreased sympathetic stimulation to the bladder and bladder neck, resulting in relaxation of the bladder neck and unopposed facilitation of parasympathetic nerve activity
3. Bladder contraction and emptying through the open urethra

16. Children acquire cerebrocortical control, which allows them to inhibit or initiate voiding.

17. Estrogen helps maintain the tone of the pelvic floor and urethral resistance. Loss of estrogen results in a loss of tone in the pelvic floor and decreased urethral resistance.

18. The prostate gland contributes to urethral resistance, which supports continence. If the gland hypertrophies, urethral obstruction may lead to retention of urine.

19. Older adults are more prone to incontinence because of neurologic changes that affect the ability to effectively inhibit voiding, and because of physiologic changes (prostate hypertrophy in men; loss of estrogen in women).

REFERENCES

1. Barrington FJF: The nervous mechanism of micturition, Q J Physiol 8:33, 1914.
2. Bradley WE, Timm GW, and Scott FB: Innervation of the detrusor muscle and urethra, Urol Clin North Am 1:3, 1974.
3. Caine M and Raz S: The role of female hormones in stress incontinence. Presented at the 16th Congress of Societé Internationale d'Urologie, Amsterdam, 1973.
4. Clegg EJ: The musculature of the human prostatic urethra, J Anat 91:345, 1959.
5. DeGroat WC and Kawatani M: Neurologic control of the urinary bladder, J Neurourol Urodyn 4:285, 1985.
6. DeGroat WC et al: Organization of the sacral parasympathetic reflex pathways to the urinary bladder and large intestines, J Auton Nerv Syst 3:135, 1981.
7. Downie JW: The autonomic pharmacology of the urinary bladder and urethra: a neglected area, Trends Pharm Sci 2:163, 1981.
8. Elbadawi A: Neuromorphologic basis of vesicourethral function. I. Histochemistry, ultrastructure, and function of intrinsic nerves of the bladder and urethra, J Neurourol Urodyn 1:3, 1982.
9. Elbadawi A and Schenk EA: Dual innervation of the mammalian urinary bladder: a histochemical study of the distribution of cholinergic and adrenergic nerves, Am J Anat 119:405, 1966.
10. Elmer M, Alm P, and Kullendorff CM: Innervation of the child urinary bladder, Scand J Urol Nephrol 20:267, 1986.
11. Gosling J: The structure of the bladder and urethra in relation to function, Urol Clin North Am 6:31, 1979.
12. Kuru M: Nervous control of micturition, Physiol Rev 45:425, 1965.
13. Maggi CA and Meli A: Review: the role of neuropeptides in the regulation of the micturition reflex, J Auton Pharmacol 6:133, 1986.
14. Ouslander JG: Lower urinary tract disorders in the elderly female. In Raz S, ed: Female urology, Philadelphia, 1983, WB Saunders Co.
15. Resnick NM and Yalla SV: Aging and its effect on the bladder, Semin Urol 5[2]:82, 1987.
16. Resnick NM, Yalla SV, and Laurino E: The pathophysiology of urinary incontinence among institutionalized elderly persons, N Engl J Med 320[1]:1, 1989.

17. Siroky MB and Krane RJ: Neurologic aspects of detrusor sphincter dyssynergia, with references to the guarding reflex, J Urol 127:953, 1982.
18. Tanagho EA: Anatomy of the lower urinary tract. In Walsh PC, Gillenwater RF, and Perlmutter AD, eds: Campbell's urology, Philadelphia, 1986, WB Saunders Co.
19. Tapp AJS and Cardozo LD: The post-menopausal bladder, Br J Hosp Med 35:20, 1986.
20. Walter JS et al: Urethral responses to sacral stimulation in the chronic spinal dog, Am J Physiol, 1990, (in press).
21. Wear JB: The neurogenic bladder. In Kendall AR and Karafin L, eds: Urology, Philadelphia, 1983, Harper & Row, Publishers, Inc.
22. Yalla SV et al: Functional striated sphincter component at the bladder neck: clinical implications, J Urol 118:408, 1977.
23. Zinner NP, Sterling AM, and Ritter RC: Structure and forces of continence. In Raz S, ed: Female urology, Philadelphia, 1983, WB Saunders Co.

2 Pathophysiology of Urinary Incontinence

JERRY G. BLAIVAS
LESLIE OLIVER

JERRY G. BLAIVAS
LESLIE OLIVER

OBJECTIVES

1. Identify the three categories of voiding dysfunction according to Wein.

2. Describe the conceptual basis for each of the following classification systems for voiding dysfunction:
   Wein classification system
   North American Nursing Diagnosis Association (NANDA) classification system
   Gray-Dougherty classification system

3. Describe key events in the micturition cycle.

4. Identify the symptoms commonly associated with involuntary detrusor contractions (bladder instability).

5. Identify three known causes of involuntary detrusor contractions (bladder instability).

6. Describe the treatments for patients with involuntary detrusor contractions, including the indications, advantages, and disadvantages of each.

7. Explain how reduced bladder compliance affects the patient's long-term health and renal function.

8. Explain how the patient with poor bladder compliance is best treated and monitored.

9. Identify the treatment options for patients with incontinence related to fistula formation.

10. Describe the two pathophysiologic mechanisms that result in stress incontinence.

11. Define the following terms:
   Type 0 stress incontinence
   Type 1 stress incontinence
   Type 2 stress incontinence
   Type 3 stress incontinence
   Sphincteric incontinence

12. Identify treatment options for patients with the following:
   Stress incontinence caused by pelvic descent (type 0 to type 2)
   Type 3 stress incontinence
   Sphincteric incontinence

13. Explain the pathophysiology of detrusor areflexia.

14. Identify the treatment options for patients with urinary retention related to reduced detrusor contractility.

15. Identify the most common cause of bladder outlet obstruction.

16. Explain the objective of treatment for patients with bladder outlet obstruction.

17. Explain detrusor-external sphincter dyssynergia (DESD), including the following:
   Pathophysiology
   Effects on bladder and sphincter function
   Potential for upper urinary tract (renal) damage

18. Differentiate type 1, type 2, and type 3 sphincter dyssynergia by the degree of urethral obstruction in each case.

19. Identify treatment options for patients with DESD.

CLASSIFICATION SYSTEMS FOR VOIDING DYSFUNCTION

The function of the urinary bladder is the storage and timely expulsion of urine. The classification system described by Wein[22] provides a simple and practical view of voiding dysfunction. Wein classified voiding dysfunctions as (1) storage problems, (2) emptying problems, and (3) combinations of storage and emptying problems. The box on p. 25 shows the Wein classification system in more detail.

Several other systems of classification are currently used to describe urinary incontinence. The three classification systems used in this text are the Wein schema, the North American Nursing Diagnosis Association (NANDA) classification system, and the Gray-Dougherty schema of pathophysiologic mechanisms. Table 2-1 provides a comparison of these classification systems.

CLASSIFICATION OF VOIDING DYSFUNCTIONS[22]

I. Storage problems
  A. Because of the bladder
    1. Involuntary detrusor contractions
      a. Detrusor instability (idiopathic, benign prostatic hypertrophy [BPH])
      b. Detrusor hyperreflexia (suprasacral neurologic lesion)
    2. Low bladder compliance
      a. Neurogenic (myelodysplasia)
      b. Fibrotic (indwelling catheter, tuberculosis [TB])
    3. Sensory urgency
      a. Infection or inflammation or both
      b. Tumor
    4. Fistula
  B. Because of the sphincter
    1. Stress incontinence
    2. Sphincteric incontinence
II. Emptying problems
  A. Because of the bladder
    1. Detrusor areflexia
    2. Impaired detrusor contractility
    3. Psychogenic retention
  B. Because of the outlet
    1. Prostatic obstruction
    2. Urethral obstruction (strictures, valves)
    3. Vesical neck obstruction
III. Storage and emptying problems
  A. Detrusor-external sphincter dyssynergia
  B. Bladder outlet obstruction combined with involuntary detrusor contractions

Table 2-1 Comparison of classification systems for voiding dysfunction

NANDA (North American Nursing Diagnosis Association)	WEIN (storage/emptying)	Gray-Dougherty (pathophysiologic mechanisms)
Stress incontinence	Storage problem (sphincter incompetence)	Stress incontinence
Urge incontinence	Storage problem (involuntary detrusor contraction)	Instability incontinence (sensation intact)
Reflex incontinence	Storage and emptying problems	Instability incontinence (loss of sensation)
Urinary retention	Emptying problem	Paradoxical/overflow incontinence
Total incontinence	Storage problem	Extraurethral incontinence
Functional incontinence	Storage problem	No separate category (functional components considered with all types)

NORMAL MICTURITION
Micturition Cycle

To understand voiding dysfunction the nurse must understand the normal cycle of micturition. The cycle begins when the bladder receives urine through the ureters. As the bladder slowly fills with urine, the pressure inside the bladder remains low. When the detrusor muscle reaches a certain threshold of distention (the micturition threshold), sensory nerve endings in the bladder wall are stimulated to transmit the sensation of fullness (the need to urinate) to the spinal cord through the pelvic nerve; other nerves then transmit this message to the brain. The brain then sends messages back down the spinal cord and out through peripheral nerves to initiate voiding (at an appropriate time and place). This sequence of events is known as the micturition reflex.[9,11]

The normal sequence of events in voiding (the micturition reflex) is characterized by (1) relaxation of the external sphincter, (2) a rise in detrusor pressure and a fall in urethral pressure, (3) opening of the vesical neck, and (4) urinary flow. Fig. 2-1 shows a normal micturition reflex as it appears on a cystometrogram (CMG).

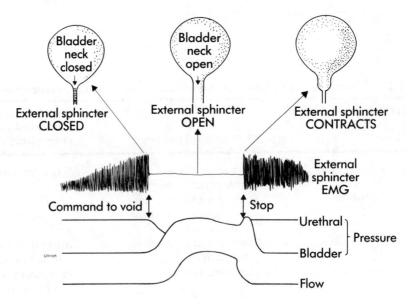

Fig. 2-1   Sequence of events during normal micturition: external urethral sphincter relaxes and urethral pressure falls, just before detrusor contraction. During voiding, entire proximal urethra is isobaric with bladder. (From Blaivas JG et al: Ann NY Acad Sci, 436, 1984.)

Effect of Neurologic Lesions on Micturition

Normal bladder function depends on intact neural pathways. Interruption of either the sensory or the motor pathways affects bladder function.

The sacral portion of the spinal cord contains the sacral micturition center (S2-4). The sacral micturition center is housed within the conus medullaris, which begins at about the level of the first lumbar vertebra. Injuries at or below this level usually result in an areflexic bladder, whereas injuries above this level cause a hyperreflexic bladder.[20]

STORAGE PROBLEMS CAUSED BY BLADDER ABNORMALITIES
Involuntary Detrusor Contractions

Characteristics. Involuntary detrusor contractions (detrusor instability, uninhibited contraction) are the most common cause of storage problems. In this condition the bladder contracts involuntarily during filling. Normally the bladder does not contract unless the patient is trying to void; urination is under voluntary control. The symptoms most commonly associated with involuntary contractions are urinary frequency, urgency, and urge incontinence.

A simple CMG usually demonstrates the presence or absence of involuntary contractions. Fig. 2-2 illustrates both a voluntary detrusor contraction (Fig. 2-2, *A*) and an involuntary (unstable) contraction (Fig. 2-2, *B*). On a CMG, voluntary and involuntary contractions appear similar; both contractions are of approximately the same height, and both produce urine flow. Sometimes the patient is trying to urinate (Fig. 2-2, *A*), sometimes not (Fig. 2-2, *B*). The only way to distinguish between voluntary and involuntary contractions is to ask the patient whether he or she is trying to void.

Patients with involuntary detrusor contractions may perceive the contraction as an urge to void; once aware of the contraction, some patients are able to abort the contraction by contracting the external urinary spincter and thus maintain continence until they reach the bathroom. Others are unable to abort the contraction and are incontinent. Still others are completely unaware of the contraction and simply void uncontrollably. The ability to abort involuntary contractions can be assessed during a CMG by asking the patient (during an involuntary contraction) to try to stop urinating. If the CMG shows a rapid return to baseline pressure at this point, it usually indicates that the patient is able to abort the contraction.

Involuntary detrusor contractions are not volume dependent, that is, they may occur with any amount of urine in the bladder. This explains why some patients have symptoms of urgency and leakage of small amounts of urine shortly after voiding. Uninhibited bladder contractions may occur sponta-

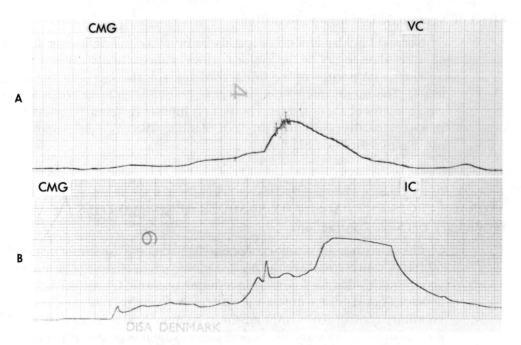

Fig. 2-2 **A,** Voluntary detrusor contraction. **B,** Involuntary detrusor contraction. The only way to distinguish between voluntary and involuntary contractions is to ask patient whether he or she is trying to void.

neously or may be provoked by such maneuvers as rapid bladder filling, alterations in posture, and coughing. During a CMG, rapid bladder filling may be seen to evoke an involuntary contraction.

Causes. Bladder instability may be caused by obstruction of the bladder outlet, inflammation of the bladder, neurologic conditions that affect the ability to inhibit bladder contractions, or unknown factors.

Bladder outlet obstruction. One cause of uninhibited contractions is bladder outlet obstruction. Urodynamic studies of patients with outlet obstruction resulting from benign prostatic hypertrophy (BPH) frequently reveal involuntary bladder contractions; these patients commonly have the symptoms of frequency, urgency, and urge incontinence that are typical of bladder instability.

Inflammatory bladder conditions. Uninhibited contractions may also result from an inflammation of the bladder wall: bladder infection, stones, environmental irritants, and tumors are possible causes of inflammation. Inflammation increases the irritability of the detrusor muscle, which causes involuntary contractions.

Neurologic conditions that cause loss of inhibition. As explained previously, normal voiding is controlled voluntarily by the cerebral cortex. With normal cerebrocortical function, voiding can be delayed; the frontal cortex sends inhibitory messages to the pontine micturition center and the bladder.[2] Neurologic lesions that damage the cortex (such as stroke, multiple sclerosis, and Parkinson's disease) commonly cause the loss of this "ability to inhibit" and result in involuntary contractions and incontinence. Involuntary contractions caused by neurologic lesions are termed "detrusor hyperreflexia."

Idiopathic bladder instability. Some patients have involuntary contractions (bladder instability) for which there is no discernible cause. In these situations the detrusor instability is termed "idiopathic."

Treatment. Effective treatment of involuntary contractions is directed toward eliminating etiologic factors and controlling the incontinence.[14]

Eliminating etiologic factors. If the patient has only a storage problem (incontinence resulting from involuntary contractions, with the bladder emptying normally), therapy is directed toward eliminating the involuntary contractions. In contrast, for the patient with involuntary detrusor contractions associated with obstruction of the bladder outlet, therapy must relieve the obstruction.[9] (Eliminating the involuntary contractions without relieving the underlying obstruction is likely to result in urinary retention.)

For the patient with inflammation of the bladder, eliminating irritants is an obvious first step in treatment. Treating an infection, eliminating stones or tumors, reducing or eliminating environmental irritants such as caffeine or bath preparations, or a combination of these steps may be necessary.

Controlling unstable contractions. Medications, behavior modification (toileting programs), biofeedback therapy, electrical stimulation, or combinations of these may be used to control involuntary contractions.

Anticholinergic and antispasmodic medications may be used to reduce the contractility and irritability of the bladder. These agents reduce the symptoms of frequency, urgency, and urge incontinence and may increase bladder capacity (by reducing bladder contractility). Medications are not necessarily the best treatment. Some patients are unable to tolerate the side effects of a particular drug and must discontinue its use before an effective dose is reached. Even medications that are well tolerated and effective do not correct the underlying disease, they simply control symptoms: when the medication is discontinued, the involuntary contractions and the urge incontinence return.

Many patients with involuntary contractions (instability incontinence, urge incontinence) benefit from behavioral therapy (behavior modification programs) designed to increase the patient's control of bladder function. Such programs combine instruction in exercises that strengthen the pelvic floor with gradual increases in the time between voidings (the voiding interval). Patients are asked to keep voiding diaries that document the time and intensity of each urge to void and the time and the amount of urine at voiding. One advantage of behavioral therapy is that patients are taught to regain control of bladder function; since the therapy addresses the underlying dysfunction, it is usually effective even after the treatments have been discontinued. However, effective behavioral therapy takes time and motivation; patients must understand that improvement is gradual and that the success of the therapy depends on their motivation and compliance with the program.

Biofeedback therapy is sometimes used to teach patients pelvic floor exercises. The strength of a muscle contraction is measured and recorded, and the information is displayed so that the patient can "see" how well he or she is contracting a particular muscle. Electrical stimulation of the sphincter muscle is also used to control unstable contractions. Exercises that strengthen the pelvic floor (with or without biofeedback therapy) and electrical stimulation are effective because repeated contraction of a muscle strengthens its tone and contractility. In addition, contraction of the pelvic floor muscles inhibits detrusor muscle contractility; this is a reflex response to pelvic floor muscle contraction.

Low Bladder Compliance

Characteristics and Causes. Reduced compliance of the bladder wall causes a rapid rise in detrusor pressure as the bladder fills with urine. A pressure of more than 40 cm H_2O at bladder capacity is considered diagnostic of low compliance (Fig. 2-3). Low compliance may be caused by any condition that leads to fibrosis of the bladder wall (such as multiple bladder operations or chronic indwelling catheter). Low compliance may also result from neurologic conditions that affect neural pathways (for example, myelodysplasia) or from surgical procedures resulting in inadvertent injury to the pelvic nerves (for example, radical hysterectomy or abdominoperineal resection of the rectum).

Treatment. Without proper treatment, low compliance of the bladder wall usually leads to damage of the upper urinary tract. Patients are usually treated

Fig. 2-3 Poor compliance, characterized by steep rise in intravesical pressure during filling. End filling pressure in this patient is 90 cm H_2O.

with clean intermittent catheterization performed often enough to ensure that intravesical pressure remains low. Since patients are unable to tell whether their filling pressures are high or low, patients with low compliance must be seen regularly (to monitor filling pressures and ensure that they remain at safe levels).

Sensory Urgency

Unknown Origin. Sensory urgency is a severe urge to void at low bladder volumes in the absence of involuntary detrusor contractions.[1] Urologic evaluation of patients with sensory urgency of unknown origin usually reveals normal cystoscopic findings and negative results of urinalyses and urine cultures. Results of CMGs usually reveal stable bladders, but patients describe intense urgency or pain at low bladder volumes. Patients seldom have incontinence, although they describe symptoms of severe frequency, urgency, and suprapubic or vaginal pain. Currently the most effective treatment for these patients is behavior modification.

Urinary Tract Infection. Sensory urgency and frequency may also result from urinary tract infections. Nonspecific infections of the genitourinary tract are usually caused by aerobic, gram-negative enteric rods (for example, *Escherichia coli*); those infections acquired outside a hospital usually respond quickly to short-term antibiotic therapy, whereas hospital-acquired infections are usually more resistant and may require intravenous antibiotic therapy.[17]

Fistula

Fistulas can cause severe problems with the storage of urine, since they permit urine to bypass the normal urethral sphincter mechanism. The most common fistula, a vesicovaginal fistula, usually results as a complication of gynecologic surgery. With this condition there is an abnormal connection between the bladder and vagina. As the bladder fills with urine, or as the patient urinates, some of the urine follows the fistulous path and drains through the vagina instead of the urethra. Surgery is usually required to correct a fistula.

STORAGE PROBLEMS CAUSED BY SPHINCTER ABNORMALITIES
Stress Incontinence

The International Continence Society has defined stress incontinence as a symptom (involuntary loss of urine associated with sudden physical exertion such as coughing, sneezing, or exercising), a sign (the observation of urine loss during increases in abdominal pressure), and a condition (the involuntary loss of urine when, in the absence of a detrusor contraction, intravesical pressure exceeds intraurethral pressure). With this condition the amount of urine lost varies from a few drops to gushes of urine, which necessitate the use of containment products. In some patients, exertion such as coughing or exercising triggers an involuntary detrusor contraction; when this happens, the patient usually voids suddenly and uncontrollably. This condition is known as stress hyperreflexia, or stress-urge incontinence.

Pathophysiology. Stress incontinence may be caused by two different pathophysiologic mechanisms: loss of structural support to the bladder neck and proximal urethra, and intrinsic sphincter dysfunction.

Loss of structural support to bladder neck and proximal urethra. Loss of structural support to the bladder neck and proximal urethra is the most common cause of stress incontinence in the female and is caused by pelvic descent (relaxation of the pelvic floor). As explained in Chapter 1, the bladder neck and proximal urethra are normally well supported in an intra-abdominal position; this support is important to continence because any increases in abdominal pressure are transmitted equally to both the bladder and the bladder neck and proximal urethra. With loss of support (that is, pelvic floor relaxation), when intra-abdominal pressure rises, the pelvic floor descends; this descent "repositions" the bladder neck and proximal urethra *outside* the abdominal cavity (Fig. 2-4). Thus increases in abdominal pressure (such as those that occur with coughing, laughing, lifting, and the like) are transmitted to the bladder but not to the bladder neck and proximal urethra. As a result, there is a sharp increase in

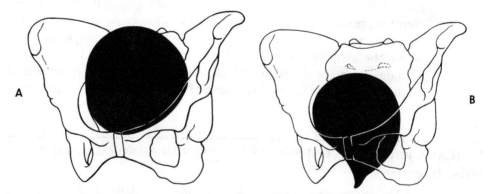

Fig. 2-4   Changes in position of bladder neck during stress maneuvers in patient with pelvic floor relaxation. **A,** At rest, base of the bladder is flat and situated above superior margin of pubic symphysis. **B,** During cough, rotational descent of urethra and bladder base occurs. (From Blaivas JG and Olsson CA: J Urol 139:727, 1988.)

intravesical pressure with no balancing increase in urethral pressure, which causes urine to leak during certain activities. The patient with stress incontinence secondary to pelvic descent is continent at rest because the sphincter mechanism itself, which is normal, maintains a urethral pressure at rest that is greater than the intravesical pressure.

Stress incontinence caused by pelvic floor relaxation can be classified as type 0, type 1, or type 2 according to the degree of pelvic descent. Videourodynamic studies may be helpful in diagnosing the particular type of stress incontinence. In type 0 stress incontinence the vesical neck and proximal urethra at rest are closed and situated at or above the superior margin of the pubic symphysis. During stress, the vesical neck and proximal urethra descend and open but no leakage occurs; leakage is probably prevented by voluntary contraction of the external sphincter. In type 1 stress incontinence, the vesical neck at rest is closed and situated at or above the inferior margin of the pubic symphysis. During stress the vesical neck and proximal urethra descend less than 2 cm and open and leakage occurs. In type 2 stress incontinence, the vesical neck at rest is closed and situated at or above the inferior margin of the pubic symphysis. During stress, the vesical neck and proximal urethra descend more than 2 cm and open; leakage occurs and a cystourethrocele is obvious.

Intrinsic sphincter dysfunction. In the second type of stress incontinence the urethra no longer functions as a sphincter. This may be caused by loss of innervation or by conditions that cause the urethra to become fibrotic or rigid.[6] Urethral pressure is usually low, and urinary leakage occurs with only minimal activity.

Intrinsic sphincter dysfunction in women is classified as type 3 stress incontinence. During bladder filling the vesical neck and proximal urethra remain open, allowing for incontinence with little provocation. For these patients, incontinence is caused not by pelvic descent but by actual loss of sphincter function.

Treatment. For women with stress incontinence, all treatment is elective and is determined by the severity of the symptoms and the degree to which they cause a patient concern or interfere with her life-style. Some women do not find it limiting to change a protective pad several times a day, whereas others find dampness after a game of golf intolerable.

A number of surgical procedures are used for the treatment of type 1 and type 2 stress incontinence. All these procedures are designed to restore the normal support for the bladder neck and proximal urethra, so that their intra-abdominal position is maintained during stress maneuvers. Commonly used procedures are further discussed in Chapter 4.

For type 3 stress incontinence, simple restoration of support is frequently ineffective. Surgical procedures that provide urethral compression are often necessary; the most common procedure is the pubovaginal sling, in which a small fascial "sling" is used to provide urethral compression. This and other treatments are further discussed in Chapter 4.

Sphincteric Incontinence

Characteristics and Causes. Urine leakage in men is referred to as sphincteric incontinence. It occurs when the urethral sphincter mechanism no longer maintains a watertight seal, so that urine leaks either because of gravity or with minimal provocation.[7] Sphincteric incontinence may be caused by surgical procedures or disease processes that lead to proximal urethral sphincter insufficiency or distal urethral sphincter denervation or both. Surgical procedures or disease processes that may impair sphincter function include abdominoperineal resection of the rectum, prostatectomy, radical hysterectomy, and pelvic radiation therapy.

Incontinence may occur after prostatectomy because the proximal urethral sphincter is removed during this procedure. Since continence after a prostatectomy depends on the distal urethral sphincter, preservation of this sphincter is essential for postoperative continence.[12]

Treatment. The man with urinary leakage requires a thorough evaluation of voiding function. Treatment options for the patient with sphincteric incontinence include an artificial urinary sphincter implantation, periurethral injections of Teflon or collagen, pharmacologic paralysis with clean intermittent catheterization, or combinations of these. These treatments are further discussed in Chapter 4.

EMPTYING PROBLEMS CAUSED BY BLADDER ABNORMALITIES

Incontinence may result from conditions that cause urinary retention; in such cases, incontinence occurs when the bladder becomes so overfilled that urine leaks out. This type of incontinence has been labeled "paradoxical incontinence."

Detrusor Areflexia

Characteristics and Causes. The absence of a detrusor contraction during a CMG indicates an acontractile detrusor. Loss of contractility caused by a neurologic lesion is properly called "detrusor areflexia."

Detrusor areflexia is most commonly caused by a neurologic process or injury that affects the lumbar or sacral vertebrae. As explained in Chapter 1, the nerve fibers that innervate the bladder and sphincter mechanism exit the spinal cord at the lumbosacral level; interruption of these pathways results in a denervated (acontractile) bladder and loss of voluntary sphincter control. In most cases of areflexia the bladder neck and distal sphincter remain closed. Conditions that may result in detrusor areflexia include herniated intervertebral discs in the lumbosacral spine; diabetic neuropathy; lesions or tumors of the lumbosacral cord (including spinal cord injury); and pelvic surgery such as radical hysterectomy or abdominoperineal resection of the rectum, which can cause damage to the pelvic or pudendal nerves or both.[2] (Damage to the pelvic nerve impairs bladder contractility, whereas damage to the pudendal nerve compromises voluntary control of the external sphincter.)

Treatment. Clean intermittent catheterization is the usual treatment for patients with detrusor areflexia. Administration of pharmacologic agents may also be necessary. Treatments are further discussed in Chapter 4.

Impaired Detrusor Contractility

Characteristics and Causes. The normal bladder contracts strongly enough, rapidly enough, and long enough to empty its contents with a normal pattern of urinary flow. When detrusor contractility is impaired, the normal pattern is reversed. As Fig. 2-5 depicts, the detrusor contraction is of low magnitude (less than 29 cm H_2O) and the accompanying flow rate is low. Although diagnostic criteria have not been clearly established for this condition, a maximum detrusor pressure of 30 cm H_2O or less that is associated with a urinary flow rate of less than 12 ml/sec justifies a diagnosis of impaired detrusor contractility.[3] Impaired contractility may be caused by a neuropathy, partial denervation, or loss of muscle tone and contractility resulting from chronic distention.

Patients with impaired detrusor contractility are unable to effectively empty their bladders; symptoms usually include a weak urinary stream and a feeling of incomplete emptying. Accurate diagnosis usually requires formal urodynamic studies. A pressure-flow study as described in Chapter 3 is usually sufficient, whereas a study of the urinary flow rate alone is usually not sufficient, since it does not distinguish between a poor flow caused by obstruction and a poor flow caused by impaired contractility.

Treatment. Treatment options for these patients include toileting programs (scheduled voiding and double voiding), administration of medications, and clean intermittent catheterization programs.

Psychogenic Retention

Characteristics and Causes. Psychogenic retention usually occurs in females, the onset is usually precipitous, and the urologic history and physical exami-

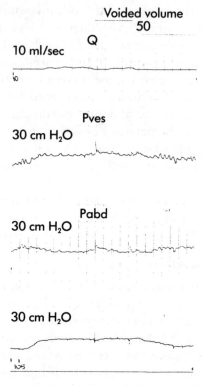

Fig. 2-5 Impaired detrusor contractility, characterized by low flow rate (5 ml/sec) and weak detrusor contraction (29 cm H_2O). (From Blaivas JG: Urology 23[5]:424, 1984.)

nation reveal no organic cause of the retention. In the assessment of these patients, care must be taken to rule out the possibility of any subtle neurologic injury. (Preminger et al.[18] found that the most common cause of urinary retention was an acute neurologic lesion, although they thought that 30% of the cases were psychogenic.)

Treatment. For these patients, intermittent catheterization is usually necessary until normal bladder function is regained.[19]

EMPTYING PROBLEMS CAUSED BY BLADDER OUTLET ABNORMALITIES

Overflow incontinence may also be caused by obstruction involving the bladder outlet; in such a case the bladder has normal contractility but distal obstruction prevents effective emptying.

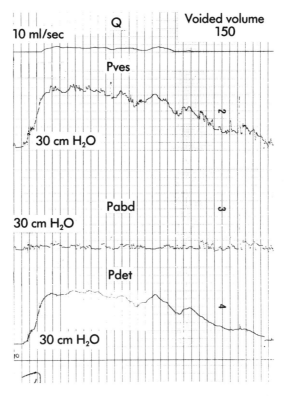

Fig. 2-6 Bladder outflow obstruction, characterized by high voiding pressure (120 cm H_2O) and low flow rate (4 ml/sec). (From Blaivas JG: Urology 32[6]:424, 1988.)

Prostatic Obstruction

Causes and Characteristics. Benign prostatic hypertrophy (BPH) is probably the most common cause of urinary obstruction in middle-aged and older men. By the age of 60 the incidence of BPH is 50%, and it increases to 80% by the age of 80.[4]

The most overt abnormality in BPH occurs when a hyperplastic prostate gland impinges on and narrows the lumen of the urethra. However, evidence suggests that there may also be a neuromuscular component to prostatic obstruction: the prostatic urethra is also narrowed by an active contraction of the smooth muscle. As the prostate grows, its increasing size causes a compression of the urethra that obstructs the outflow. Outflow obstruction is evident when a strong detrusor contraction of adequate duration and speed occurs in conjunction with a poor flow rate. The CMG tracing in Fig. 2-6 depicts a detrusor contraction of 120 cm H_2O with a maximum flow rate of 4 ml/sec.

Patients usually have both obstructive and irritative signs. They have difficulty starting the stream of urine, and they have a feeling of incomplete emptying, which may progress to complete urinary retention. Patients commonly have symptoms of frequency, urgency, urge incontinence, and nocturia, the classic signs of bladder instability (involuntary contractions).

Approximately two thirds of the patients with BPH have both detrusor instability and prostatic obstruction.[8] Transurethral resection of the prostate (TURP) usually relieves the obstruction but may or may not alleviate the involuntary contractions. After prostatectomy, involuntary contractions are eliminated in approximately 70% of the patients, although elimination may take as long as 1 year. Thirty percent of the patients have persistent involuntary contractions (p. 27), which require additional intervention.

Treatment. Currently the "gold standard" for treating the symptoms of BPH is a prostatectomy. Recently however, patients with BPH have been offered a variety of nonsurgical options including balloon dilatation, prostatic coils, microwave techniques, and experimental drugs.

Urethral Obstruction

Urethral outlet obstruction can be caused by urethral strictures and posterior urethral valves.

Urethral Strictures. Most acquired urethral strictures are caused by infection or trauma. The narrowing of the urethra that results from the stricture impedes the urinary flow. A retrograde urethrogram (RUG) or a voiding cystourethrogram (VCUG) or both will reveal the location and severity of the stricture. The obstruction may be mild and result only in frequency, or severe enough that the patient cannot void at all. Treatment options include urethral dilatation, urethrotomy, and surgical reconstruction.

Posterior Urethral Valves. Posterior urethral valves are a congenital condition found during infancy or childhood in boys. The "valves" are mucosal folds in the distal prostatic urethra that obstruct voiding. The degree of obstruction is extremely variable: boys may have mild, moderate, or severe symptoms of obstruction[21] and poor or intermittent urinary streams. Infection and sepsis may occur, and hydronephrosis has occurred in severe cases.

After diagnosis, treatment is directed toward destruction of the valves. Transurethral fulguration of the valves is usually successful in cases of mild to moderate obstruction.[13] In more severe cases a vesicostomy or cutaneous loop ureterostomies may be required for immediate diversion. In such cases reconstruction of the urinary tract is performed at a later date.[16]

Vesical Neck Obstruction

Vesical neck obstruction occurs when the vesical neck does not fully open and funnel during voiding. This condition is uncommon in men and exceedingly rare in women. The patient with vesical neck obstruction usually has the classic symptoms of obstruction (that is, difficulty starting the urinary stream, poor stream, and incomplete emptying).

STORAGE AND EMPTYING PROBLEMS

Patients with suprasacral neurologic lesions may have dysfunctional voiding patterns involving both the storage and the emptying phase of the micturition cycle.

Characteristics and Causes

Suprasacral lesions result in loss of voluntary control of voiding and loss of bladder-sphincter coordination because the pontine-sacral axis has been interrupted; however, the reflex arc between the bladder and the sacral cord is maintained. Thus the bladder contracts spontaneously, via the sacral reflex arc, at certain volumes or in response to certain stimuli. Simultaneously, the external (distal urinary) sphincter may contract because the neural pathways that control sphincter relaxation (from the brain and pons to the sacral cord and external sphincter) have been lost. This condition is known as detrusor external sphincter dyssynergia (DESD).

On clinical examination the patient has involuntary detrusor contractions at the same time that the external sphincter contracts. These patients are in essence voiding against an obstruction. DESD can be classified as type 1, 2, or 3, depending on when the sphincter contracts and relaxes (Fig. 2-7).[10] In type 1 DESD the sphincter initially contracts but then suddenly relaxes at the height of the detrusor contraction, thus allowing for unobstructed voiding. In type 2 the sphincter contracts and relaxes intermittently throughout the detrusor con-

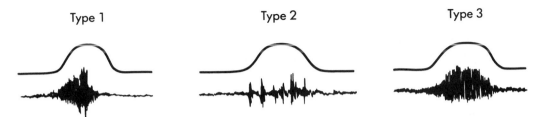

Type 1   Type 2   Type 3

Fig. 2-7   Types of dyssynergia. In type 1, EMG activity is increased during first part of detrusor contraction. At peak of detrusor contraction, there is sudden relaxation and voiding ensues. In type 2, EMG activity increases sporadically throughout detrusor contraction. In type 3, EMG activity has "crescendo and decrescendo" appearance that continues throughout detrusor contraction. (From Blaivas JG: J Urol 125:454, 1981.)

traction. In type 3 the sphincter remains contracted during the detrusor contraction; for voiding to occur, the detrusor contraction must be strong enough to overcome the urethral contraction. During such uncoordinated voiding, intravesical pressures can rise to extremely high levels; this "high-pressure" voiding leads to upper urinary tract deterioration.

Treatment

The goal of treatment is to protect the upper urinary tract by eliminating high-pressure, obstructed voiding. Several treatments are available for patients with DESD. Probably the most common is the use of anticholinergic medications to eliminate bladder contractions and clean intermittent catheterization to empty the bladder effectively. For the patient with a small bladder capacity, augmentation cystoplasty may be necessary before a catheterization program is begun.

Some patients (for example, some quadriplegics) are not candidates for clean intermittent catheterization. Men may be treated instead with external sphincterotomy and condom catheter drainage; women may need indwelling catheters (because indwelling catheters seem to cause fewer problems in women and because currently there are no suitable external collection devices for women).[15] In some cases urinary diversion may be necessary.

All patients with a combination of storage and emptying problems should be evaluated at least yearly, since these patients are at high risk for such complications as infection and bladder stones caused by urinary stasis, immobility, or pubic hairs inadvertently introduced into the bladder during intermittent catheterization.[2] An intravenous pyelogram should be performed at least once a year to check for upper urinary tract damage.

SUMMARY

Voiding dysfunctions can be classified as problems with storage (stress incontinence, instability or urge incontinence, and total incontinence), problems with emptying (paradoxical incontinence), and combined storage and emptying problems (reflex incontinence and instability incontinence). A voiding dysfunction can be further classified as either a problem involving the bladder or a problem involving the sphincter mechanism.

Problems with storage cause incontinence but do not threaten the function of the upper urinary tract unless bladder compliance is compromised. Problems with emptying and combined storage and emptying problems create a "hostile" incontinent state in which the function of the upper urinary tract is threatened. In assessment and treatment, both the incontinence and the health of the upper urinary tract must be considered.

SELF-EVALUATION

QUESTIONS

1. Identify the three categories of voiding dysfunction according to Wein.
2. Identify the terms used by the North American Nursing Diagnosis Association (NANDA) classification system and the Gray-Dougherty system to describe the following:
   a. Storage problems
   b. Emptying problems
   c. Combined storage and emptying problems
3. Explain what is meant by "involuntary contractions," or "detrusor instability."
4. List three symptoms commonly associated with instability incontinence, or involuntary contractions
5. Explain how patients can abort involuntary contractions.
6. Identify possible causes of involuntary contractions, or detrusor instability.
7. Explain what is meant by the term "idiopathic detrusor instability."
8. Identify at least two treatments for patients with involuntary contractions.
9. Explain why routine follow-up evaluation is critical for patients with storage problems resulting from low bladder compliance.
10. Sensory urgency is best treated with:
    a. Antibiotics
    b. Antispasmodics
    c. Behavior modification, or toileting programs
    d. Surgical intervention
11. Describe the two pathophysiologic mechanisms that may be involved in stress incontinence.
12. Define the following terms:
    a. Type 1 stress incontinence
    b. Type 2 stress incontinence
    c. Type 3 stress incontinence
    d. Sphincteric incontinence
13. Explain why some degree of stress incontinence in men is common after prostatectomy.
14. Treatments for patients with intrinsic sphincter dysfunction include:
    a. Artificial sphincter implantation; periurethral injections
    b. Behavioral therapy, or toileting programs
    c. Clean intermittent catheterization
    d. Antispasmodic medications
15. Detrusor areflexia most commonly results from:
    a. Loss of normal structural support to the bladder neck

b. Neurologic processes that cause loss of cerebrocortical function and loss of inhibition

c. Neurologic lesions that affect motor pathways to the bladder

d. Damage to the intrinsic sphincter mechanism

16. Patients with impaired detrusor contractility or loss of detrusor contractility are best managed by:

   a. Sympathomimetic medications

   b. Behavioral therapy, or toileting programs

   c. Artificial sphincter implantation

   d. Clean intermittent catheterization

17. Benign prostatic hypertrophy is the most common cause of bladder outlet obstruction in older men.

   a. True

   b. False

18. Patients with prostate hypertrophy are likely to seek medical advice because of symptoms of:

   a. Obstruction and instability

   b. Obstruction and sphincter incompetence

   c. Obstruction alone

   d. Detrusor areflexia

19. Explain the pathophysiology of detrusor external sphincter dyssynergia (DESD).

20. Differentiate type 1, type 2, and type 3 DESD in terms of external sphincter activity and risk to the upper urinary tract.

21. The primary goal of treatment for patients with DESD is:

   a. To protect the upper urinary tract by eliminating high-pressure, obstructed voiding

   b. To eliminate urinary incontinence

22. The most common treatment plan for the patient with dyssynergia is:

   a. Clean intermittent catheterization

   b. Behavioral modification, or toileting programs

   c. Artificial sphincter implantation

   d. Biofeedback

SELF-EVALUATION

ANSWERS

1. **a.** Storage problems
   b. Emptying problems
   c. Combined storage and emptying problems
2. **a.** Storage problems
       NANDA: stress incontinence, total incontinence, and urge inconti-
           nence
       Gray-Dougherty: stress incontinence, extraurethral incontinence, and
           instability incontinence
   b. Emptying problems
       NANDA: retention with overflow
       Gray-Dougherty: paradoxical incontinence
   c. Combined storage and emptying problems
       NANDA: reflex incontinence
       Gray-Dougherty: instability incontinence
3. Bladder contractions that are not voluntarily initiated indicate detrusor
   instability and are called involuntary contractions.
4. Frequency, urgency, and urge incontinence. Nocturia is also commonly
   reported.
5. By learning to contract the pelvic floor muscles, which increases urethral
   pressure and inhibits detrusor contractility via a negative feedback system
6. **a.** Outlet obstruction
   b. Inflammatory bladder conditions
   c. Neurologic conditions resulting in loss of inhibition
7. "Idiopathic" instability is the term used for symptoms of instability (frequency, urgency, and urge incontinence) that have no known cause.
8. **a.** Elimination of etiologic factors (outlet obstruction or inflammation)
   b. Medications (anticholinergic or antispasmodic)
   c. Behavior modification, or toileting programs
   d. Pelvic floor exercises and biofeedback
   e. Electrical stimulation of pelvic floor muscles
9. Low bladder compliance results in high intravesical pressures. Without
   proper treatment, low compliance usually leads to upper urinary tract
   damage. Since patients cannot "sense" rising intravesical pressures, they
   must be routinely monitored for adequate bladder compliance and safe
   levels of intravesical pressure.
10. **c.** Behavior modification and toileting programs
11. **a.** Loss of structural support to the bladder neck, which causes the bladder
       neck and proximal urethra to descend *out* of the abdominal cavity during

stress maneuvers. This means that increases in abdominal pressure are transmitted to the bladder but *not* to the bladder neck and proximal urethra; thus urinary leakage occurs (intravesical pressure is greater than urethral pressure).

  b. Loss of sphincter function, which may be caused by conditions that make the urethra fibrotic, or by loss of innervation. With a loss of function, the sphincter is unable to maintain sufficient urethral pressure, and leakage occurs with minimal provocation.

12. a. Type 1 stress incontinence: the bladder neck is closed at rest and is positioned at or above the inferior margin of the symphysis pubis. During stress, the bladder neck and proximal urethra descend (less than 2 cm) and open; urinary leakage occurs.

  b. Type 2 stress incontinence: the bladder neck is closed at rest and is positioned at or above the inferior margin of the symphysis pubis. During stress, the bladder neck and proximal urethra descend (more than 2 cm) and open; urinary leakage occurs, and a cystourethrocele is evident.

  c. Type 3 stress incontinence: intrinsic sphincteric dysfunction in women is called type 3 incontinence. The bladder neck and proximal urethra remain open during filling, and urine loss occurs with minimal provocation.

  d. Sphincteric incontinence: intrinsic sphincteric dysfunction in men is called sphincteric incontinence. The urethral sphincter mechanism no longer maintains a watertight seal, and urine leaks either because of gravity or with slight provocation.

13. Prostatectomy damages or removes the internal sphincter (bladder neck); continence then depends on the distal urethral sphincter.

14. a. Artificial sphincter implantation; periurethral injections

15. c. Neurologic lesions that affect motor pathways to the bladder

16. d. Clean intermittent catheterization

17. a. True

18. a. Obstruction and instability

19. Detrusor external sphincter dyssynergia (DESD) is likely to occur with suprasacral neurologic lesions. In such a case, loss of voluntary control and loss of bladder sphincter coordination is caused by interruption of the pontine-sacral axis; however, detrusor contractility is maintained via the sacral reflex arc. Because of the loss of nerve pathways that control external sphincter relaxation, the bladder may contract against a closed sphincter. This syndrome (bladder contraction with simultaneous contraction of the external sphincter) is also known as bladder-sphincter dyssynergia.

20. a. Type 1: there is initial contraction of the external sphincter, and relaxation of the sphincter occurs at the height of the detrusor contraction.

Unobstructed voiding then occurs, so type 1 poses the least risk for the upper urinary tract.

    b. Type 2: the external sphincter contracts and relaxes sporadically throughout detrusor contraction. This creates some degree of obstruction and therefore poses risk for the upper urinary tract.

    c. Type 3: the external sphincter remains contracted throughout detrusor contraction, creating high-pressure, obstructed voiding; this condition poses a *major* risk to the upper urinary tract.

21. a. To protect the upper urinary tract by eliminating high-pressure, obstructed voiding.

22. a. Clean intermittent catheterization.

REFERENCES

1. Abrams P et al: The standardization of terminology of lower tract function, Scand J Urol Nephrol [Suppl]114:5, 1988.
2. Amis ES and Blaivas JG: Neurogenic bladder simplified, Radiol Clin North Am 1990 (in press).
3. Axelrod SA and Blaivas JG: The distinction between poor detrusor contractility and bladder outlet obstruction. Proceedings of the International Continence Society, Boston, 1986.
4. Barry SJ et al: The development of human benign prostatic hyperplasia with age, J Urol 132:373, 1984.
5. Blaivas JG: Neurologic dysfunctions. In Yalla SV, McGuire EJ, Elbadawi A, and Blaivas JG, eds: Neurourology and urodynamics: principles and practice, New York, 1988, Macmillan Publishing Co.
6. Blaivas JG: Terminology and abbreviation. In Yalla SV, McGuire EJ, Elbadawi A, and Blaivas JG, eds: Neurourology and urodynamics: principles and practice, New York, 1988, Macmillan Publishing Co.
7. Blaivas JG: Pubovaginal sling. In Whitehead ED, ed: Current operative urology, Philadelphia, 1989, JB Lippincott Co.
8. Blaivas JG: Sphincter electromyography, J Neurourol Urodyn 2[4]:267, 1984.
9. Blaivas JG and Kaplan SA: Treatment alternatives in BPH, Hosp Med, 1990 (in press).
10. Blaivas JG and Olsson CA: Stress incontinence: classification and surgical approach, J Urol 139:727, 1988.
11. Cavanaugh J: How your urinary system functions. In Gartley CB, ed: A guide to living with loss of bladder control, Ottawa, 1985, Jameson Books, Inc.
12. Hadley R, Zimmern P, and Raz, S: Surgical treatment of urinary incontinence. In Yalla S, McGuire E, Elbadawi A, and Blaivas J, eds: Neurourology and urodynamics: principles and practice, New York, 1988, Macmillan Publishing Co.
13. Johnson JH and Kulatilake AE: The sequelae of posterior urethral valves, Br J Urol 43:743, 1971.
14. Katz GP and Blaivas JG: A diagnosis dilemma: when urodynamic findings differ from clinical impression, J Urol 129:1170, 1983.
15. Lloyd LK: New trends in urologic management of spinal cord injured patients: voiding dysfunction in patients with neurologic disease, AUA Home Study Course, Series XI [1]:27, American Urological Association, 1988.
16. McAninch JW: Disorders of the penis and male urethra. In Smith DR, ed: General urology, Los Altos, Calif, 1984, Lange Medical Books.
17. Meares EM: Nonspecific infections of the genitourinary tract. In Smith DR, ed: General urology, Los Altos, Calif, 1984, Lange Medical Books.
18. Preminger GM et al: Acute urinary retention in female patients: diagnosis and treatment, J Urol 130:112, 1983.
19. Smith DR: Effects of the psyche on renal and vesical function. In Smith DR, ed: General urology, Los Altos, Calif, 1984, Lange Medical Books.
20. Tanagho EA: Neuropathic bladder disorders. In Smith DR, ed: General urology, Los Altos, Calif, 1984, Lange Medical Books.
21. Uehling T: Posterior urethral valves, Funct Classif Urol 15:27, 1980.
22. Wein AJ: Classification of neurogenic voiding dysfunction, J Urol 125:605, 1981.

3 Assessment of Patients with Urinary Incontinence

MIKEL GRAY

OBJECTIVES

1. Discuss the components of a voiding habits history.
2. Identify the components of a limited review of systems and medical-surgical history as it relates to urinary incontinence.
3. Describe the relationship between abnormality of the neurologic system and urinary incontinence.
4. Explain the relationship between commonly used prescription and over-the-counter drugs and the pathophysiology of urinary incontinence.
5. Identify the components of a physical examination appropriate for the patient who seeks medical advice because of altered patterns of urinary elimination.
6. Describe the components of an assessment of the functional ability of the individual with urinary incontinence.
7. Discuss psychosocial issues relevant to the assessment of the individual with urinary incontinence.
8. Explain the relevance of the patient's cognitive function and level of motivation to the assessment and management of urinary incontinence.
9. List laboratory studies required for baseline assessment of the individual with urinary incontinence.
10. Interpret findings from a voiding diary in the assessment of the individual with urinary incontinence.
11. Interpret the significance of observing voided stream and measuring post-void residual volume in the assessment of the individual with urinary incontinence.
12. Identify indications for referral for urologic and urodynamic assessment of the individual with urinary incontinence.
13. Use assessment data to determine the type of urinary incontinence and appropriate bladder management program for an individual with urinary incontinence.

HISTORY

A thorough history is the first component in a complete assessment of a patient with incontinence. Ideally the history is obtained by oral interview. Because the oral history contains much unrelated but pertinent data, a checklist is used to facilitate adequate documentation (Fig. 3-1).

It is best to begin the interview with an open-ended statement or question that allows the person to describe those aspects of incontinence that he or she perceives to be causing problems. "Tell me about your bladder control problem" is an appropriate opening statement for the patient seeking help specifically for urinary incontinence. Patients more reluctant to discuss a bladder control problem may be asked, "Are you having any problems with urination or bladder control?" The interviewer then explores the duration of any problem with leakage. Occasionally an individual seeks medical advice because of incontinence caused by an acute problem such as urinary tract infection or calculi. More often, however, the problem represents a chronic condition that has led to significant alterations in patterns of daily living.

After this introduction the interviewer moves through a structured set of questions to elicit data pertinent to voiding patterns and urologic history related to incontinence, as well as data concerning the patient's neurologic, reproductive, and gastrointestinal systems, related medical disorders, surgical history, and current medications.

Patterns of Urinary Elimination and Bladder Management

The individual's patterns of urinary elimination and bladder management are assessed. Every person employs some "program" or strategy to manage urinary elimination. Clearly, most people spontaneously void to evacuate urine, but some are forced to adopt alternative strategies.

Diurnal and Nocturnal Voiding. If the person voids spontaneously, the interviewer determines patterns of diurnal and nocturnal elimination. The questions, "How often do you urinate during the day?" or "How many times do you urinate while you are awake?" rarely elicit an accurate assessment. It is more effective for the interviewer to encourage the individual to describe an interval of time between trips to the bathroom. For example, the patient may be asked if he or she could sit through a two-hour movie without emptying the bladder, or asked to estimate how often during a long drive he or she must stop to urinate. The normal pattern is to urinate no more often than every 2 hours during waking hours. Excessive urinary frequency indicates sensory urgency disorder, bladder instability, or urinary retention.

The interviewer assesses nocturnal patterns of urinary elimination by asking the person how many times he or she rises to void during sleep. Nocturia occurs

Voiding history

Bladder management program   Diapers _____   Pads (no. per day) _____

Intermittent catheterization   Frequency q _____ hours

Indwelling catheter _____

Spontaneous voiding   Diurnal frequency q _____ hours

Nocturia (times per night) _____

Stream   Explosive   Normal   Intermittent   Poor or dribbling

Straining   Crede

Incontinence   Stress   Urge   Reflex   Overflow   Constant   Functional

Sensations   Normal   Diminished or Absent

Retention   Acute   Chronic   Feelings of incomplete emptying

Urologic history

Cystitis   Current   Chronic   Recurrent

Febrile urinary tract infections (UTIs):   Yes   No

Other _____

Neurologic history

Spinal cord injury (_____)   Parkinsonism   Alzheimer's

Seizure disorders   Traumatic brain injury   Cerebrovascular accident (stroke)

Other _____

Related medical conditions

Diabetes _____   Cancer _____

Other _____

Bowel habits   Constipation   Incontinence

Pattern _____   Usual consistency _____

Reproductive system of man

Benign prostatic hypertrophy   Prostatitis   Prostate cancer

Erectile dysfunction   Ejaculatory dysfunction

Reproductive system of woman

Number of vaginal deliveries _____

Forceps assist _____   Other: _____

_____

Surgical history

Current medications

Fig. 3-1   Checklist used to summarize and document pertinent information obtained from patient history.

when an individual is waked from sleep by the desire to void. The interviewer helps the patient determine whether it is the urge to urinate that causes the waking, or other factors. One episode of nocturia each night is considered normal, and elderly individuals may waken as often as twice each night without associated voiding dysfunction.

Containment Devices. Some individuals who spontaneously void also wear a urine containment device such as a pad to cope with incontinence. The nurse should ask these patients what type of product they wear and how often it is changed. This information gives some indication of the severity and frequency of incontinence; however, a person's economic status, sense of hygiene, and fear of embarrassment also affect how often the product is changed. For example, some patients are greatly bothered by even a small amount of leakage and wear particularly heavy or absorbent pads to protect themselves from embarrassment; as soon as the pads become wet, these patients are likely to change to dry ones. In contrast, a less fastidious or economically comfortable patient may wear a single pad until it becomes thoroughly soaked or dampens clothing.

Some individuals have such severe urinary leakage that they must use a diaper either to contain leakage between spontaneous voidings or to contain all urinary output. The interviewer must determine how long the patient has used diapers to manage leakage and what elimination patterns led to their use.

Indwelling Catheter. Some people manage their bladders by wearing indwelling catheters. The interviewer should attempt to determine why a catheter was first used and how long a catheter has been worn. When considering a bladder management program for the patient with an indwelling catheter, the nurse must determine whether the person is willing to remove the catheter and try another program (such as intermittent catheterization) or whether he or she simply wishes to keep the catheter and prevent leakage around the tube.

Intermittent Catheterization. Some patients manage urinary elimination by intermittent catheterization. The interviewer should determine the *prescribed* as well as the *actual* schedule of catheterization. For example, the interviewer may ask the patient to describe a typical day and to identify the times when he or she would be likely to catheterize. This inquiry may be followed by the standard question, "How often do you catheterize?" The patient is likely to answer this question by describing whatever regimen the primary caretaker or urologist recommends, regardless of the actual frequency of catheterization.

Fluid Intake. After patterns of urinary elimination are assessed, the interviewer determines the patterns of fluid intake. The individual may be asked to describe the types and amounts of fluids he or she consumes during a typical day (24-hour period). Specifically, the patient is asked to estimate both the volume of water and clear juices consumed and the volume of caffeinated fluids and citrus juices consumed. The interviewer should also ask the individual to correlate the volumes and types of beverages consumed with urinary frequency and the likelihood of leakage. Many individuals associate the consumption of caffeine or citrus juices with heightened sensations of urgency and frequency; reducing or eliminating the consumption of such beverages may be indicated.

Patterns of Incontinence

Once the bladder management program and patterns of urinary elimination have been determined, the patient is asked to describe his or her patterns of incontinence. As stated in Chapter 2, several schemas are used to classify incontinence by symptoms or pathophysiologic mechanisms (see Table 2-1). The interviewer should learn and consistently use one of these schemas to classify the historical description of leakage into one or more types of incontinence. In this chapter, two classification systems are used: the schema based on pathophysiologic mechanisms as described by Gray and Dougherty[10] and the schema now used by the North American Nursing Diagnosis Association (NANDA)[3] (see Table 2-1).

Stress Incontinence. Stress incontinence occurs when physical exertion produces urinary leakage. The degree of stress incontinence ranges from mild to severe. The patient is asked whether leakage occurs with coughing, sneezing, or heavy lifting. Leakage that occurs only with physical exertion is a symptom of mild to moderate stress incontinence. Patients with severe stress incontinence report that leakage occurs whenever they assume an upright position or engage in any form of physical exertion, no matter how slight; this condition is classified by NANDA as total incontinence. Stress incontinence is distinguished from urge incontinence by the fact that leakage is *not* associated with a sense of urgency to urinate.

Instability Incontinence. Instability incontinence is classically defined as "contraction of the bladder without its owner's permission" that results in urinary leakage. In other words, involuntary detrusor contractions cause the leakage. NANDA has classified instability incontinence as either urge incontinence or reflex incontinence.[3]

Urge incontinence. The symptom produced when bladder instability occurs in an individual who has intact sensory function of the lower urinary tract is urge incontinence. The patient often describes episodes of precipitous urination and inability to reach a toilet "in time." The individual should be asked whether warning signs precede incontinent episodes. Typically, the person reports a sense of urgency just before or at the beginning of urinary leakage.

Reflex incontinence. The pattern produced when bladder instability occurs in an individual who does not have normal sensations in the lower urinary tract is reflex incontinence. The most common cause of reflex incontinence is a lesion or disease of the spinal cord that produces an unstable bladder with loss of pelvic sensations.[10] The patient may state that he or she "reflexes" or that the bladder empties itself at unpredictable times. Some patients can stimulate micturition by stroking the suprapubic area or inner thigh or by pulling pubic hair; however, they are unable to voluntarily initiate or inhibit voiding. Because sensations of filling are diminished or absent, these patients often describe atypical warnings of impending micturition, such as tingling in the legs or abdomen. Some patients are not aware that they are voiding until they perceive urine leaking onto their skin.

Some individuals with lesions of the thoracic or cervical spinal cord may notice headache, dizziness, or flushing immediately before and during episodes of reflex incontinence. These sensations are caused by excessive stimulation of the sympathetic nervous system. This condition, called *autonomic dysreflexia,* is diagnosed by monitoring blood pressure, which rises precipitously when bladder contractions occur. It represents a serious associated dysfunction that requires prompt management.[13]

Overflow (Paradoxical) Incontinence. Overflow or paradoxical incontinence occurs when symptoms of dribbling or leakage are caused by an inability to effectively empty the bladder. NANDA classifies this condition as urinary retention.[8] The person with overflow incontinence commonly reports urinary frequency and nocturia, as well as dribbling or leakage. Often the patient is aware of incomplete bladder emptying and feels only partial relief after micturition. Patients with long-term urinary retention lose sensations of bladder filling; such patients report symptoms of frequent urination and nocturia but deny feelings of incomplete bladder emptying.

Continuous (Extraurethral) Incontinence. Continuous or constant urinary leakage occurs when congenital or acquired anatomic defects cause urine to bypass the normal sphincter mechanism. NANDA classifies this type of urine loss as total incontinence. Typically patients describe a complete loss of the ability to store urine. Some patients have both normal spontaneous voiding and continuous dribbling that is not associated with urgency or physical exertion (for example, patients with vesicovaginal fistula).

Functional Incontinence. NANDA uses the term "functional incontinence" to describe urinary leakage caused by environmental or functional factors. Cognitive deficits or motivational disorders produced by organic brain disorders or mental health disorders may result in functional incontinence. (The interviewer should ask family members or caretakers to supplement the patient's history, if cognitive or communicative deficits render the patient an unreliable historian.) There is no pathophysiologic diagnosis that correlates to the NANDA diagnosis of functional incontinence; this is because functional incontinence is not associated with any pathologic condition of the urinary system or voiding mechanism (see Table 2-1). *Any* type of incontinence can be exacerbated by functional factors. For example, the instability (urge) incontinence of a 68-year-old woman may be made worse by such functional and environmental factors as arthritis, decreased mobility, and a long distance to the bathroom.

Characteristics of Urinary Stream

Once the type of incontinence has been determined, the force and character of the urinary stream are assessed. The patient is asked to describe the stream, and the interviewer attempts to classify it as adequate (normal), explosive, intermittent, or poor.

Normal Stream. The normal urinary stream begins within 15 seconds of an attempt to initiate voiding. The diameter of a normal stream is approximately that of a pencil lead; the stream is expressed continuously until the person feels that the bladder is completely emptied. The person should not have to strain to maintain the stream and should be able to interrupt micturition on command. The stream should not spray at the urethral meatus or form an arc several feet in front of the male. A normal urinary stream indicates effective bladder emptying but does not rule out the possibility of abnormalities in bladder filling and storage.

Explosive Stream. The explosive urinary stream may or may not be associated with urgency to void. The patient typically describes an explosive stream as particularly forceful and brief. The patient usually does not have to strain to produce an explosive stream and may not be able to interrupt the stream on command. The explosive stream is often associated with stress incontinence resulting from reduced outlet resistance, but in females it may be normal.

Intermittent Stream. The intermittent stream is usually accompanied by straining. The patient often states that the stream stops before he or she feels "finished" with micturition and that he or she must strain or wait several minutes before completing micturition. The intermittent stream may be accompanied by urgency to void or by hesitancy in initiating micturition; often it is associated with feelings of incomplete bladder emptying and with postvoid dribbling. An intermittent stream may indicate bladder outlet obstruction or compromised detrusor contractility.

Poor Stream. The patient with a poor urinary stream usually notices a decrease in the force of the stream; many patients strain to increase its force. Men with bladder outlet obstruction and a poor stream often describe sensations of adequate pressure despite a poor urinary flow, as if they were voiding "through a dam." Urinary hesitancy often is associated with poor urinary stream; when outlet obstruction is complicated by bladder instability, urgency may also occur. A prolonged postvoid dribble typically occurs in men with poor urinary stream and prostatic obstruction. A poor urinary flow may also be caused by inadequate detrusor contractility.

Sensations of Bladder Filling

After evaluating the patient's urinary stream, the interviewer assesses the patient's sensations of bladder filling. The patient is asked to place his or her index finger in the area where the greatest sensation of bladder fullness is produced. A female with normal filling sensations usually indicates the urethral or vaginal area; she places her finger on the clitoris, vaginal opening, labia, or urethral meatus, and she may describe the sensation of bladder fullness as a tickle. A male with normal sensations usually points to the urethral meatus, glans, or dorsal aspect of the penis, and he too is likely to describe the sensation of fullness as a tickle.

Patients with diminished sensations of bladder filling usually describe bladder fullness as a pressure (rather than a tickle) that is centered over the pubic symphysis or the lower abdomen. Patients with absent sensations often state that they feel no sensations or that they determine the need to urinate by watching the time or by noticing leakage.

Focused Review of Systems and Medical-Surgical History

Assessment of urinary incontinence should include evaluation of the patient's urologic, neurologic, reproductive, sexual, and bowel function; the patient's medical and surgical history must be reviewed, and medications the patient has taken or is taking must be assessed. A focused review of systems for the patient with urinary incontinence is outlined in the box on the following page. When questioning patients about urinary function, the interviewer must remember that many people do not distinguish one structure of the urinary tract from another. For example, a patient may refer to the entire genitourinary tract as "my kidneys." By asking general questions about the urinary tract, the interviewer often elicits information about various urologic conditions; such

FOCUSED REVIEW OF SYSTEMS

I. Urologic system
  A. Urinary tract infection
    1. Lower urinary tract infection (cystitis)
    2. Upper urinary tract infection (pyelonephritis)
    3. History of vesicoureteral reflux
  B. Urinary tract tumors and stones
  C. Renal insufficiency
  D. Other urinary tract problems
II. Neurologic system
  A. General indicators of dysfunction (motor-sensory loss)
  B. Central nervous system
    1. Lesions
      a. Tumor
      b. Stroke
      c. Multiple sclerosis
      d. Others
    2. Organic diseases
      a. Alzheimer's disease
      b. Others
    3. Trauma
    4. Surgical procedures
  C. Spinal cord
    1. Injury
      a. Vertebral level
      b. Extent of involvement
    2. Lesions and conditions
      a. Multiple sclerosis
      b. Transverse myelitis
      c. Others
  D. Peripheral nervous system
    1. Back conditions and treatments
    2. Peripheral neuropathy
      a. Symptoms
      b. Associated medical conditions
        (1) Diabetes mellitus
        (2) Others
III. Reproductive system
  A. Female
    1. Number of vaginal deliveries
    2. Obstetric complications or difficult deliveries
    3. Gynecologic conditions
      a. Vaginitis
      b. Sexually transmitted diseases
      c. Others
    4. Premenopausal or postmenopausal status
    5. Symptoms of pelvic floor relaxation
  B. Male
    1. Prostate disorders
      a. Benign prostatic hypertrophy (BPH)
      b. Prostatitis
      c. Tumor
      d. Others
    2. Reproductive infections
      a. Sexually transmitted diseases
      b. Epididymo-orchitis
      c. Others
    3. Erectile function
    4. Ejaculatory function
IV. Gastrointestinal system
  A. Frequency of bowel movements
  B. Typical stool consistency and caliber
  C. Patterns of bowel control
V. General medical history
  A. Chronic conditions being treated
    a. Diabetes mellitus
    b. Hypertension
    c. Cancer
    d. Others
  B. Sensory disorders
    a. Loss of vision
    b. Hearing loss
    c. Others
VI. Surgical history
VII. Pharmacologic assessment
  A. Prescription drugs
    a. Reason for prescription
    b. Duration of use
  B. Over-the-counter drugs
    a. Reason for use
    b. Duration of use

information contributes to a more thorough history of the patient's incontinence. The interviewer should ask open-ended questions and follow up any clues presented.

Occasionally assessment reveals a condition that requires prompt referral. For example, any patient with a voiding dysfunction and suspect neurologic findings should be referred to a urologist (or another physician).

PHYSICAL EXAMINATION

The history is followed by a limited physical examination designed to elucidate specific findings pertinent to the assessment and management of the patient with incontinence. The physical examination includes a limited assessment of the patient's nervous system, an assessment of fine and gross motor movements, and inspection of the genitalia and adjacent integument.

Neurologic Examination

Mentation and Motivation. The examiner begins by assessing the patient's general state of mentation: the patient's hygiene, the appropriateness of clothing for current weather conditions, and the patient's general alertness are observed. The patient's motivation and interest in altering behaviors to cope with incontinence are also assessed. If the patient's family or caregiver has answered questions throughout the review of the patient's history, the examiner should then directly assess the patient's orientation to time, place, and person. This assessment may be followed by *simple* questions that require quantitative analysis (that is, counting or simple addition) and abstract reasoning (such as the interpretation of an analogy or a simple story).[15] These assessments of a patient's cognitive status and motivational level are critical to establishment of an effective bladder management program.

Motor Skills. Motor skills are assessed by observing the patient as he or she manipulates clothing and removes undergarments in preparation for the examination of the genitalia. The examiner notices the type of clothing the patient wears, the condition of the clothing, and the skill and speed with which the patient manipulates zippers, buttons, belts, shoelaces, or Velcro material. This information is valuable when the nurse attempts to improve the patient's dexterity and speed when toileting. Balance may be assessed by administering the Romberg test, in which the patient is asked to stand with feet together and arms at the side, first with eyes open and then with eyes closed. Gait is assessed by asking the patient to walk several paces and noticing the use of aids such as a walker or a cane.[15] This assessment of motor skills is crucial to attempts to improve the patient's mobility and access to bathroom facilities.

Back and Lower Extremities. After the patient has removed his or her clothing and put on an appropriate gown, the examiner inspects the patient's feet for signs of clubbing, which may indicate congenital spinal abnormalities. In addition, the lower back and buttocks are inspected for signs of spinal dysraphism such as a lipomatous area, hairy tuft, or skin tag over the lower back. The examiner evaluates the lower extremities for obvious signs of muscular asymmetry or differences in muscle strength that may indicate neurologic abnormality.

This limited neurologic examination is completed during the assessment of the genitalia and related integument, which is discussed in the following section.

Genitalia and Related Integument

Female. Signs of estrogenization of the vaginal mucosa, signs of pelvic descent, and the appearance of the urethral meatus are assessed.

Estrogenization of vagina and meatus. The examiner locates the urethral meatus, which is normally pink and assumes an ovoid shape. The urethral mucosa normally resembles a rosebud because of the redundancy of the mucosal lining. In the estrogen-deficient woman, the meatus may appear thinned and may have lost its characteristic pink color. The vaginal mucosa is then inspected; it is normally pink, rugated, and moist. The estrogen-deficient vaginal mucosa may lose its color, appear dry, and be tender to touch.

Signs of pelvic descent. Inspection of the vaginal vault for signs of pelvic descent is reserved for clinicians trained in the use of a vaginal speculum. The examiner chooses an appropriately sized speculum and detaches the inferior blade from the top portion of the speculum. After positioning the patient and explaining the procedure to her, the examiner places two gloved fingers into the vaginal introitus and applies gentle downward pressure; the woman is asked to breathe slowly and deeply and to relax the circumvaginal muscles.[15] Once the examiner detects relaxation of the circumvaginal muscles, the inferior blade of the speculum is lubricated and inserted into the vaginal vault at a 45-degree angle. After the blade is positioned against the posterior vaginal wall, the woman is asked to bear down by using the abdominal muscles. Bulging of the bladder into the anterior vaginal wall indicates a cystocele. The speculum is then gently rotated to rest against the anterior vaginal wall and the maneuver is repeated; bulging of the rectum into the vault indicates a rectocele. The speculum is then nearly removed and the patient is again asked to strain the abdominal muscles. This procedure allows the examiner to detect vaginal prolapse, which appears as descent of the cervix toward the vaginal introitus. Pelvic descent correlates with but is not diagnostic of stress urinary incontinence.

Perineal skin. The perineal skin is inspected for lesions or loss of integrity caused by urinary leakage. When leakage is continuous or frequent, a red maculopapular rash with satellite lesions (consistent with fungal infection) is commonly found, as is ammonia contact dermatitis.

Perineal sensation and bulbocavernosus muscle response. The neurologic examination of the genitalia is completed by assessing local sensations and the bulbocavernosus response (BCR). The BCR is assessed by gently inserting a lubricated, gloved finger into the rectum. The tone of the anal sphincter is assessed during insertion, and the finger is left in place. The other hand is used to tap the clitoris or, when an indwelling catheter is in place, to place gentle traction against the bladder neck. A positive BCR occurs when stimulation produces tightening of the anal sphincter around the finger; this response indicates a grossly intact neural pathway between the pelvic floor muscles and sacral roots. A negative BCR associated with abnormal anal sphincter relaxation may indicate denervation. Before removing the finger, the examiner asks the patient to tighten the anal sphincter; this maneuver allows the examiner to assess volitional control of the pelvic floor muscles, which is mediated by the pyramidal tracts.

Male

Penis and scrotal contents. The examination begins with an inspection of the penis and scrotal contents. The examiner also assesses the skin overlying the perineal area for lesions, rashes, or loss of integrity caused by urinary leakage. The scrotum is gently palpated to detect the testes and signs of infection.

Rectum and prostate. The examiner first prepares the patient by explaining the procedure and then gently inserts a lubricated, gloved finger into the rectum. The tone of the anal sphincter is assessed, and the prostate gland is palpated. The normal prostate is firm but not hard, is approximately the size of a chestnut, and has two distinct symmetric halves (palpable lobes). In the case of benign prostatic hypertrophy (BPH), the examiner feels a bilateral, "boggy" enlargement without hardened areas. Cancer of the prostate is typically evident as one or more hardened areas in either lobe or as an area of induration; one lobe is often larger than the other. Chronic inflammation of the prostate produces bilateral tenderness with "boggy," mildly enlarged lobes. The acutely inflamed prostate is not amenable to palpation because of associated pain and the risk of systemic spread of the infection.[15] Enlargement of the prostate caused by BPH or cancer is correlated with but not diagnostic of outlet obstruction and urinary retention.

Bulbocavernosus response. After palpating the prostate, the examiner completes the neurological examination by assessing the BCR. With a finger still in the rectum, the examiner gently squeezes the glans penis. A positive response is evident when the sphincter contracts around the examiner's finger; this response indicates intact neural pathways between the sacral roots and the pelvic floor muscles. Abnormal anal relaxation and a negative BCR may indicate denervation. Before removing the finger, the examiner asks the patient to contract the anal sphincter; this maneuver permits the examiner to assess volitional control of the pelvic floor muscles, which is mediated by the pyramidal tracts.

ENVIRONMENTAL ASSESSMENT

An assessment of the patient with urinary incontinence should include an inspection of the home environment. The examiner may begin by inspecting the patient's bathroom, its lighting and flooring, obstacles such as rugs on the floor, and the presence or absence of supportive bars or handles. Lighting in the bathroom should be adequate, and a night light is recommended for patients with nocturia. The floor should not be particularly slick or cluttered with objects such as space heaters or waste baskets that may cause a fall. Rugs that slide easily on the floor should not be used. The examiner determines whether the door frame is wide enough to provide access for the individual who uses an assistive device such as a walker, wheelchair, cane, or crutches. The examiner evaluates the height and location of the toilet and its accessibility for transfers from a wheelchair.

The distance of the bathroom from other key locations in the home (sleeping, eating, and living areas) is determined. Ideally, the toilet is convenient to the living area or the place where the individual spends the most time. The examiner looks for elements in the person's environment that impede access to the bathroom, such as dimly lit passageways, slick floors, loose rugs, or stairs.

When a home visit is not feasible, an environmental checklist is completed by the patient or caregiver. The checklist is designed to include the details previously discussed.

VOIDING DIARY

A voiding diary is a valuable tool used to document information about patterns of urinary elimination. It is used in the initial assessment of incontinence and may be used again to evaluate the effectiveness of a bladder management program. The diary serves several purposes, including the assessment of diurnal and nocturnal voiding and incontinence patterns. More detailed diaries may be used to document behavioral or environmental factors that precipitate or alleviate leakage. Selection of a voiding diary is guided by considerations of the type of information sought, the motivation and knowledge of the person completing the record, and the type or types of dysfunctional voiding being documented.

The diary may be kept by the patient or the patient's caretakers or by nursing staff; it is placed near the bathroom or bedside to facilitate prompt documentation. An effective diary may be kept for only a short time: keeping a diary for 2 to 3 days provides a solid baseline of information; 4 to 7 days of documentation may provide even more detailed data. When a voiding diary is kept for too long, the patient or caretaker may become tired and frustrated and the accuracy of data is often reduced.

It is essential to discuss results of the document with the patient and participating caregivers after the diary has been completed. This discussion provides an opportunity to elucidate details of a proposed bladder management program and to reinforce the importance of an accurate voiding diary in the assessment and ongoing management of incontinence.

Selection of Voiding Diary

The simplest voiding diary documents only the patterns of urinary elimination (Fig. 3-2). It typically contains two columns; the patient records the time and then places a check mark or an *x* in one column each time he or she voids and in the other column each time he or she leaks urine or discovers leakage. This diary is used to assess diurnal and nocturnal voiding patterns, as well as patterns of urinary incontinence. It is easily kept by patients at home, and little expertise or judgment is required to accurately complete the record.

In a more sophisticated diary the recorder documents the volume of urine voided, as well as the time at voiding (Fig. 3-3). The patient or recorder is given a graduated beaker, graduated urinal, or "high hat" urine collector. For as long as the diary is being kept, the patient voids only into the collection device. Because it is difficult to estimate the volume of leakage, incontinence is recorded only as a check mark. The patient or recorder is usually asked to maintain the diary for 2 to 3 days or for no longer than 1 week.

Voiding diaries may also include estimates of the volume of fluids consumed (Fig. 3-3). Since it is unrealistic to expect the patient outside the hospital setting to measure all fluid intake, these diaries usually rely on estimates of volume consumed. A table of estimates of fluid volumes (for example, coffee cup = 6 oz) is included with the diary.

Other diaries are tailored for the hospital or inpatient environment (Fig. 3-4). These diaries are maintained for longer periods of time to provide continual assessment and evaluation of bladder management programs. To ensure completeness of documentation for extended periods of time, the information required is limited to the volume of urine voided, the time at voiding, and "check mark" documentation of incontinence episodes.

Voiding diaries may be used to evaluate both behavioral and environmental factors associated with voiding and incontinence. These diaries usually provide a space for comments, and the incontinent individual or caregiver is asked to

Time	Sunday		Monday		Tuesday		Wednesday		Thursday		Friday		Saturday	
	Voided	Leaked	Voided	Leaked	Voided	Leaked	Voided	Leaked	Voided	Leaked	Voided	Leaked	Voided	Leaked

Fig. 3-2 Simple voiding diary. Patient records time and places check mark in appropriate column when he or she voids and when urine leakage is noted.

Time	Amount voided	Leakage	Amount of fluid consumed

Fig. 3-3   More detailed voiding diary that documents voiding patterns, volume of urine voided, and estimates of volume of fluid consumed.

describe circumstances surrounding leakage (for example, urgency, altered mental or emotional status, problems with mobility, or activity associated with the leakage). The success of this type of diary is significantly influenced by the motivation and knowledge of the patient or record keeper.

Interpretation of Data

Interpretation of the voiding diary is influenced by how long the diary is kept, what information it provides, and the completeness and accuracy of the recorded data. A discussion of findings with the patient or caregiver when the diary is returned also yields valuable information concerning patterns of urinary elimination, leakage, and the probable accuracy of the recorded data.

Patterns of Urinary Elimination. The voiding diary provides a relatively accurate log of patterns of urinary elimination. First, the nurse determines the patient's usual patterns of sleep and wakefulness. The nurse never assumes that the patient is awake in the morning and asleep during the night and early

Shepherd Spinal Center
Treatment Administration Record

					Pg.	of	

Date	INI	Treatment	Time		Date in.	Date in.	Date in.	Date in.	Date in.
ord.		Bladder Program		I.C.					
				Reflex					
				Foley/Void					
d.c.				I.C.					
				Reflex					
ord.				Foley/Void					
				I.C.					
d.c.				Reflex					
				Foley/Void					
				I.C.					
				Reflex					
				Foley/Void					
				I.C.					
				Reflex					
				Foley/Void					
				I.C.					
				Reflex					
				Foley/Void					

Fig. 3-4 Inpatient voiding diary. Diary often is kept for prolonged period of time to assess urinary elimination patterns and evaluate bladder management program. (Copyright Shepherd Spinal Center, Atlanta.)

morning hours, since work requirements or other factors may profoundly alter patterns of sleep and wakefulness. The frequency of waking, or diurnal, urinary elimination is determined by noting the longest and shortest intervals between trips to the bathroom, the intervals between micturition episodes in a given day, and the average length of time between voiding episodes. Normal voiding intervals are at least 2 hours long and should be no longer than 4 to 6 hours except during sleep. Variance from these norms (as documented in a voiding diary) establishes the diagnosis of urinary frequency or infrequent voiding pattern.

Patterns of nocturia are calculated by counting the number of times the patient documented voiding during sleeping hours and dividing this number by the number of nights during which data was recorded. The average number of times per night that the patient voided is then used to assess the patient's nocturnal voiding pattern. To differentiate true nocturia from incidental voiding at night, the nurse must determine whether it was the urge to urinate that woke the patient.

Patterns of Urinary Leakage. Patterns of urinary incontinence are calculated by counting the number of times the person recorded being aware of leakage and by correlating the occurrence of wetness with events of daily living. For example, the person with stress incontinence may have documented that leakage occurred during periods of activity and exercise, whereas the person with bladder instability and urge incontinence may have recorded patterns of leakage associated with increased fluid consumption or "provocative" maneuvers (such as changing position or placing the hands in warm water). Persons with urinary retention and overflow incontinence often document particularly frequent urination and leakage during sleeping hours, when they assume a supine or prone position. In contrast, persons who experience extraurethral or continuous incontinence record that the frequency or general magnitude of leakage is unaffected by changes in position or activity levels.

When the voiding diary includes documentation of voided volume, the examiner assesses the amount of urine voided per day and the functional capacity of the bladder. The daily volume of urine voided is calculated by adding all volumes voided during a 24-hour period. The 24-hour urinary output may vary from 1000 ml to 2500 ml, depending on how much fluid was consumed and how much was lost as sweat or through the feces. The examiner should determine the reason for volumes of urine voided that are consistently high or low for a 24-hour period.

Volume and Patterns of Fluid Consumption. Assessment of excessively low or high volumes of urine voided during a 24-hour period is facilitated by documentation of the quantity of fluid consumed. For example, the person with urgency and instability incontinence may purposely restrict fluid intake in an attempt to reduce the frequency of urination and the risk of urge incontinence without realizing that this maneuver increases the risk of urinary tract infection. In contrast, frequency of urination, urgency, and nocturia may be caused by excessive water intake (water intoxication) or by diabetes insipidus and may not be a primary voiding dysfunction.

The assessment of fluid consumption is completed by correlating patterns of fluid intake with patterns of urination and incontinence. This process often provides valuable clues to the cause of incontinence and may suggest solutions to problems in bladder management. For example, the person with frequent nocturnal urination may unwittingly consume a large amount of fluid just before bedtime, thus increasing the likelihood of nocturia, or the individual with instability incontinence may consume large amounts of beverages during mealtimes, thus triggering postprandial intensification of frequency and urge incontinence.

Bladder Capacity. Bladder capacity is assessed by three methods. *Anatomic capacity* is the volume of urine the bladder is capable of holding at the limit of the muscular and vesicoelastic properties of its wall. Anatomic capacity is determined during cystourethroscopy by filling the bladder while the patient is anesthetized or sedated. Anatomic capacity is usually greater than functional capacity because sedation eliminates sensations of urgency, which normally serve to prevent overdistention. *Cystometric capacity* is the amount of urine the bladder holds during urodynamic assessment. Cystometric capacity is influenced by the rate of filling, the patient's anxiety related to testing, and the tester's clinical judgment. Cystometric capacity is often less than functional capacity.

Functional capacity is the volume of urine that can be stored in the bladder before sensations of urgency provoke the individual to seek the bathroom or before an unstable contraction causes incontinence. Functional capacity is determined by interpreting the voiding diary. The examiner determines the lowest and highest volumes of urine recorded and the average volume of urine stored before micturition. In adults the functional bladder capacity varies from 300 to 600 ml; in children the functional capacity of the bladder is estimated by using the following equation: Capacity (ml) = (Age in years + 2) × 30.

Behavioral and Environmental Factors that Influence Continence. As discussed previously, an assessment of precipitating factors is made by reviewing the data contained in a completed voiding diary. Nonetheless, in certain cases, such as when functional incontinence is suspected, a voiding diary that allows more sophisticated evaluation of factors associated with leakage is indicated (Fig. 3-5).

The voiding diary that documents functional and environmental aspects of incontinence and patterns of urinary elimination is kept by nursing staff, who must assess the patient's voiding patterns every 2 hours. Usually the patient is offered a urinal or assisted to the toilet. The results are then recorded, including the volume of urine voided and evidence of incontinence. Space is also provided for comments about the patient's behaviors and cognitive awareness of the timed voiding program. The data recorded in this diary allows the nurse to assess patterns of urinary elimination and incontinence; it also suggests the feasibility of a timed voiding program for the patient with compromised sensation, mobility, or mentation that causes functional incontinence.[4,14]

Name _____   Date _____

Time toilet is offered	Leakage (yes or no)	Was patient aware of urge? (yes or no)	Did patient void? (yes or no)	Comments
0800				
1000				
1200				
1400				
1600				
1800				
2000				

(2200 and so forth)

Fig. 3-5   Voiding diary that evaluates functional and environmental aspects of incontinence. To keep diary, nursing staff must prompt patient to void every 2 hours.

Use of Diaries in Bladder Management Programs

Voiding diaries also provide valuable information when intermittent catheterization is used in a bladder management program. These diaries document catheterized volumes and patterns of leakage (Fig. 3-4). They may be used to assess spontaneously voided volume versus residual volume obtained by catheterization (Fig. 3-6). This information is particularly valuable when a bladder management program is being determined for the patient with urinary retention; it allows ongoing assessment of the catheterized volume versus spontaneously voided volume. This information permits alteration in the catheterization schedule as indicated.

LABORATORY STUDIES
Urine Studies

Urinalysis and urine culture are part of the routine investigation of the incontinent patient. Urinalysis measures the specific gravity and the levels of

Name _____   Date _____

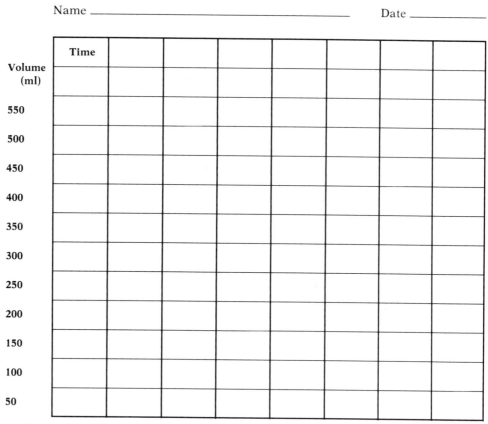

Instructions: Use a red pen to record catheterized volumes. Use a blue pen to record voided volumes.

Fig. 3-6   Voiding diary that compares catheterized volumes with voided volumes provides data that indicate when patient's intermittent catheterization schedule must be adjusted.

glucose, protein, hemoglobin, white blood cells, bacteria, and red blood cells in the urine.[17] This information helps the examiner identify factors that may precipitate incontinence (for example, diabetes insipidus, diabetes mellitus, infection, or bladder tumor) and provides clues to renal function.

Any evidence of urinary tract infection necessitates a urine culture and sensitivity. Treatment of an infection is rarely enough to ablate incontinence caused by bladder instability that is exacerbated by bacteriuria. More commonly, infection represents a complication of voiding dysfunction; it may or may not represent evidence of a serious underlying medical condition. Determining the implications of abnormal urinalysis results or urine culture indicative of infection is in the purview of the physician or urologist, and prompt consultation is indicated.

Serum Studies

When assessing any patient with incontinence, the clinician must remain constantly aware that urinary leakage is a symptom of an underlying condition. In certain instances, incontinence is a symptom of a mechanical or structural defect of the genitourinary system and carries no particular risk to health other than the considerable social and hygienic consequences of leakage. In other instances, however, incontinence is the presenting symptom of a significant obstructive uropathy or neurologic disease, and further investigation and intervention are imperative. Therefore serum laboratory values that reflect upper urinary tract function (that is, blood urea nitrogen [BUN] levels and creatinine levels) should be obtained routinely. An elevated BUN level may represent compromised renal function; elevation of the serum creatinine level represents a loss of at least 50% of functioning nephrons.[17] When BUN levels and serum creatinine levels are elevated, prompt consultation with a urologist and complex urodynamic studies are necessary to assess bladder function and its effect on the upper urinary tract.

IMAGING STUDIES

Imaging studies such as radiographs, ultrasonography, and radionuclide studies are used to evaluate the anatomic and physiologic impact of incontinence on the function of the urinary system. Imaging studies are particularly helpful in the assessment of urinary incontinence because they provide clues to compromised function of the upper urinary tract long before serum laboratory values become abnormal.

Radiographic Studies

The *plain abdominal film* of the kidneys, ureters, and bladder (KUB) is obtained by making a posteroanterior roentgenogram of the abdomen from the pubic symphysis to the thorax above the renal shadows. In the assessment of urinary incontinence the KUB serves two purposes: (1) evaluation of the renal shadows and approximate ureteral course, to identify evidence of radiopaque calculi and (2) examination of the lumbosacral spine, to identify previously undetected spinal abnormalities that may influence voiding function.[9]

An *intravenous pyelogram* (IVP) or an *intravenous urogram* (IVU) provides a detailed assessment of the renal collecting system and ureters.[9] The IVP is valuable in the assessment of urinary incontinence associated with hematuria, infection, or evidence of urinary retention indicating potential obstruction.

The *cystogram* and *voiding cystourethrogram* (VCUG) provide detailed views of the bladder and urethral anatomy and are performed by infusing contrast material into the bladder in a retrograde manner. The VCUG is the more thorough examination; it combines cystography with urethrography during micturition. The cystogram reveals bladder trabeculation or diverticula that may result from high-pressure voiding with obstruction or detrusor instability. Vesicoureteral reflux is detected and graded by the cystogram and VCUG. The VCUG allows evaluation of the urethra during micturition and reveals the location of any bladder outlet obstruction. The VCUG is most valuable in the assessment of urinary incontinence when the VCUG and the physiologic data in a *videourodynamic study* are considered together.

Ultrasonography

Ultrasonography provides a mechanism for evaluation of the upper and lower urinary tracts of the incontinent patient. Ultrasound of the upper tract reveals calculi or enlargement of the collecting system, which may indicate obstruction or vesicoureteral reflux. Ultrasound also allows qualitative assessment of the renal parenchyma without exposing the patient to radiation. Ultrasound of the lower urinary tract provides data regarding the contour and thickness of the bladder wall; structural defects such as ureterocele or diverticula can be identified. Ultrasound is also used as a noninvasive method to estimate postvoid residual urine volume.

Radionuclide Studies

Radionuclide studies may provide additional clues during the investigation of incontinence. The *diethylenetriamine pentaacetic acid (DTPA) scan* uses a radionuclide excreted by the kidney to evaluate glomerular filtration. When furosemide (Lasix) is injected during the DTPA scan, analysis of the washout of radionuclide from the kidneys provides an assessment of obstruction of the upper urinary tract. The *dimercaptosuccinic acid (DMSA) scan* uses a radionuclide that is filtered at the glomerulus and concentrated in the renal tubule. The portion that concentrates in the renal tubule allows accurate evaluation of differential renal function and identification of focal renal scars or areas in the renal parenchyma where functioning nephrons have been destroyed and replaced by fibrous tissue.[6]

Radionuclide scans are also valuable in the investigation of incontinence when dysfunctional voiding states compromise upper urinary tract function. The DTPA scan, for example, reveals obstruction long before compromised renal function causes an increase in BUN levels and creatinine levels in the serum. The DTPA scan may also detect obstruction before changes are noticeable on the IVP.[6] The DMSA scan is particularly valuable when voiding dysfunction is associated with vesicoureteral reflux and focal areas of renal scarring are suspected, or when the relative contribution of each kidney to total renal function is questioned.

URODYNAMIC STUDIES

The term "urodynamics" refers to a group of tests that measure the transport, storage, and elimination functions of the urinary tract. Urodynamic assessment allows comprehensive evaluation of bladder filling, including capacity, sensation, compliance, and detrusor stability. Urodynamic assessment during micturition evaluates detrusor contractility, urinary flow, striated sphincter response to voiding, and the relationship between pressure and flow at a given volume. Urethral pressure studies provide an assessment of urethral closure pressure, the maintenance of closure during physical exertion or stress, and the transmission of intravesical pressure across the urethral outlet during filling and micturition. Urodynamic testing is enhanced by the combination of physiologic and morphologic data obtained during the videourodynamic study. Although not every patient requires urodynamic evaluation, access to urodynamic testing is essential for the clinician who gives care to patients with incontinence.

Uroflowmetry

Uroflowmetry, or the urinary flow test, is an objective measure of the rate and force of bladder evacuation. It is completed *before* detailed urodynamic examination is undertaken. The test is noninvasive; it is easily performed and simple to interpret. Accurate evaluation requires that the patient void with a full bladder: the individual is usually asked to come to the testing situation with a moderate to strong desire to urinate. He or she is asked to void into a special device that measures urinary flow rate as milliliters per second. The patient is provided with privacy during testing to prevent inhibition of micturition caused by anxiety. Postvoid residual measurement may be undertaken via either catheterization or ultrasonic scanning.

Uroflowmetry serves two purposes in the assessment of the incontinent individual; (1) it serves as a screening study for urinary flow, and (2) it is used as a quality control measure to which data from the analysis of pressure and flow are compared.

Data from the flow study are displayed as numbers and as a chart (Fig. 3-7). Flow is represented in urodynamic terminology as "Q" and the "Qmax" represents the maximum or peak flow. The "Qave" represents the average or mean flow, which is calculated as volume divided by time in seconds. In addition, both voiding time and voided volume are determined. Postvoid residual volume may also be determined and provides valuable adjunct information.

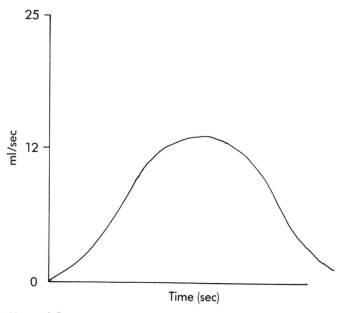

Fig. 3-7   Normal flow pattern with Qmax of 12 ml/sec and Qave of 8 ml/sec.

The graphic data is displayed as a flow "curve," which falls into one of four characteristic patterns. Interpretation of results requires evaluation of both numeric and graphic data.

Normal Flow Pattern. The normal flow pattern resembles a bell curve that may be slightly skewed to the left (Fig. 3-7). The maximum or peak flow is greater than 12 ml/sec, and the mean or average flow exceeds 8 ml/sec. In the adult the voided volume should exceed 250 ml and the residual volume is expected to be less than 100 ml, or 25% of total bladder volume.

A normal flow pattern implies that the individual empties his or her bladder efficiently and completely; however, it does not rule out the possibility of abnormalities in bladder filling and storage such as instability incontinence.

Explosive Flow Pattern. The explosive flow pattern represents a variant of normal; it is steeper than the normal pattern, with a briefer voiding time (Fig. 3-8). The Qmax and Qave values are greater than those in the normal pattern, and the voiding time is less. An explosive flow pattern is often seen in cases of stress urinary incontinence, although it *is not* diagnostic of the condition. In women an explosive flow pattern may represent a variant of normal, unobstructed voiding.

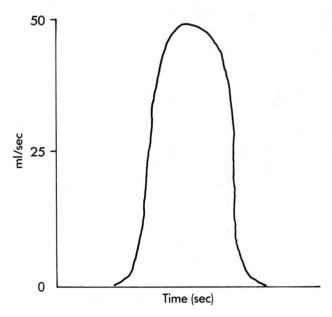

Fig. 3-8   Explosive flow pattern with Qmax of 40 ml/sec and Qave of 30 ml/sec.

Intermittent Flow Pattern. The intermittent flow pattern is characterized by a sawtooth configuration (Fig. 3-9). The Qmax, or maximum flow, is often within the normal range (more than 12 ml/sec), although the Qave or mean flow is less than 8 ml/sec. The voiding time is prolonged, the voided volume varies, and significant residual volume may be evident. An intermittent flow pattern indicates the presence of deficient detrusor function (compromised bladder contractility) or bladder outlet obstruction caused by anatomic or functional factors. Pressure-flow analysis is required to determine which of these factors is causing the intermittent flow pattern.

Poor Flow Pattern. The poor flow pattern is a depressed curve with low peak values and mean flow values (Fig. 3-10). The Qmax is less than 12 ml/sec, and the Qave is less than 8 ml/sec. The voiding time may be prolonged and volume voided may be small. Postvoid residual volumes often exceed 25% of total bladder capacity. A poor flow pattern implies the presence of bladder outlet obstruction or deficient detrusor function. Pressure-flow analysis is required to determine which of these conditions is causing the poor flow pattern.

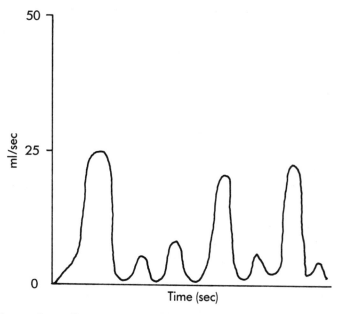

Fig. 3-9 Intermittent flow pattern with Qmax of 12 ml/sec and Qave of 4 ml/sec.

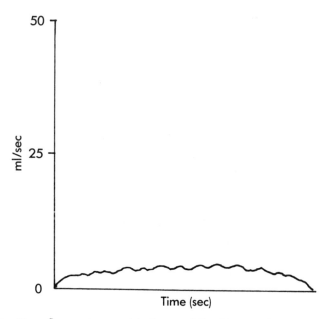

Fig. 3-10 Poor flow pattern with Qmax of 5 ml/sec and Qave of 3 ml/sec.

Detailed Assessment (Full Urodynamics and Cystometrics)

More detailed urodynamic studies often are required to discern the dynamic characteristics of urinary incontinence. Although the choice of urodynamic studies depends on the patient's presenting symptoms, assessment routinely includes a cystometrogram (CMG), an electromyogram (EMG) of the striated sphincter, and pressure-flow analysis.

Cystometrogram. The CMG provides assessment of the bladder's filling and storage function. It is a graphic representation of bladder pressure compared to volume.

Procedure. The study requires catheterization; liquid is instilled in a retrograde manner. During filling the patient is asked to report sensations of filling, and the study is terminated when the patient perceives a sensation of fullness or when unstable contractions produce premature bladder evacuation.

Sterile water, a saline solution, or water-soluble radiographic contrast material is commonly used to fill the bladder. Carbon dioxide is rarely used to fill the bladder. Gas cystometry is *not* recommended by the Urodynamics Society or the International Continence Society, since the physical characteristics of gas do not approximate the characteristics of urine as closely as do those of liquid media. The CMG is most accurate when two catheters (or a single multilumen catheter) are placed in the bladder. Typically, one tube is used to measure intravesical or total bladder pressure (Pves). A rectal tube or intravaginal balloon device is used to provide simultaneous measurement of abdominal pressure (Pabd) during bladder filling and evacuation.

A polygraph or computer used to record cystometric results provides three measurements from the CMG. Pves represents the sum of pressure placed against the bladder contents. There are two sources of this pressure: the detrusor muscle produces pressure via smooth muscle bundles in the bladder wall, and the abdomen produces pressure from adjacent muscle and external sources (gravity and the like). Simultaneous determination of Pabd and Pves allows subtraction of abdominal influences on intravesical pressure and estimation of influence on bladder pressure (Fig. 3-11). The resulting measurement is the detrusor pressure (Pdet), which represents that portion of intravesical pressure produced by detrusor contractility during bladder filling and evacuation.

Interpretation. The filling CMG is interpreted within the context of four concepts: capacity, sensation, compliance, and stability.

CAPACITY

Cystometric bladder capacity is determined by the patient's subjective reports and by the clinician's judgment (Fig. 3-12). Generally, cystometric capacity is recorded either as the volume at which the patient feels a sense of bladder fullness or when an unstable contraction causes early emptying. Cystometric bladder capacity in adults ranges from 300 to 600 ml. In infants cys-

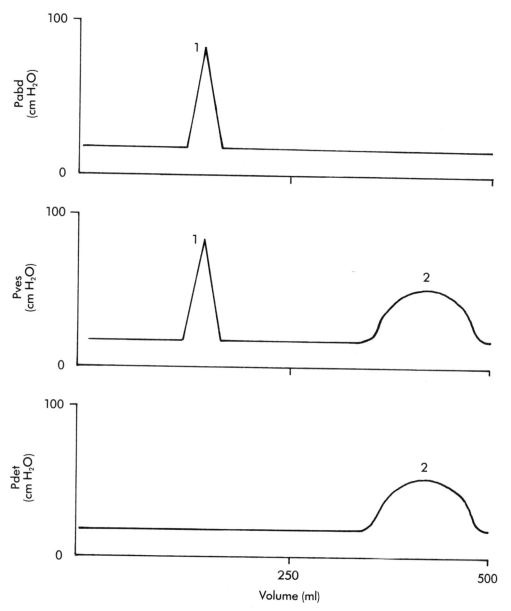

Fig. 3-11   Filling CMG with three pressure channels: *Pves* represents sum of abdominal pressure and detrusor pressure. *Pabd* is estimated by placing fluid-filled balloon in rectum. *Pdet* is electronic subtraction of abdominal pressure from vesical pressure. Difference between abdominal straining, *1*, and bladder contraction, *2*, is evident.

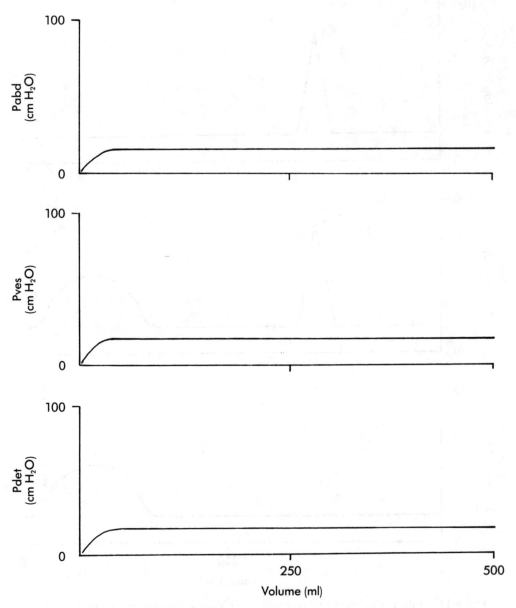

Fig. 3-12 Normal filling CMG. Relatively flat line assessed by detrusor pressure channel indicates good bladder wall compliance.

tometric capacity is approximately 15 to 60 ml. In children the equation, Capacity (ml) = (Age in years + 2) × 30, is used to estimate cystometric capacity. Cystometric capacity is often slightly less than functional capacity.

Abnormally small cystometric capacity is caused by sensory urgency or by detrusor instability. Bladder hypersensitivity is caused by an irritant disorder that inflames the bladder wall, causing decreased tolerance to filling. Bacterial or parasitic urinary tract infection, chemotherapy, and radiotherapy-induced cystitis or interstitial cystitis all cause sensory urgency with reduced cystometric capacity. Bladder calculi or tumors also cause irritation and inflammation of the bladder wall with compromised capacity. Detrusor instability provoked by bladder filling is also associated with small capacity.

Abnormally large cystometric capacity is typically the result of a loss of sensation of bladder filling. Complete absence of the sensations of filling is commonly observed with spinal cord lesions caused by trauma, disease states such as multiple sclerosis or transverse myelitis, or congenital defects such as spina bifida and myelomeningocele. Diabetes mellitus is commonly associated with impaired sensations of filling, as is chronic overdistention of the bladder caused by infrequent voiding.[10]

SENSATION

The sensations of bladder filling represent a subjective report provided by the patient. They are affected by the patient's level of anxiety and desire to please the examiner. Usually the first sensation of bladder filling and the sensation of bladder fullness are reported. In addition, sensations of urgency may be provoked by the occurrence of unstable contractions that may or may not be associated with urinary leakage. In the adult the first sensation of bladder filling normally occurs at a bladder volume of 90 to 150 ml, and the sensation of fullness occurs at a volume of 300 to 600 ml.

Abnormally early sensations indicate an irritative bladder disorder or marked anxiety; reassurance and repeated filling studies help the urodynamicist distinguish between these factors. Abnormally delayed sensations of filling indicate chronic overdistention of the bladder or partial sensory loss resulting from peripheral neuropathy or idiopathic causes. Total absence of sensations of filling usually indicates spinal cord abnormality.

COMPLIANCE

Bladder wall compliance is determined by measuring the change in vesical pressure during a change in volume. Normally the bladder fills at a relatively low pressure across a wide variance in volume. The relationship between volume and pressure in the bladder is described by the application of Laplace's law, Pdet = $F/\pi R^2$, in which *Pdet* represents detrusor pressure, *F* represents force, and *R* is radius. During passive filling, F and R tend to increase at a proportional rate, thus tending to cancel one another out. As a result, the slope

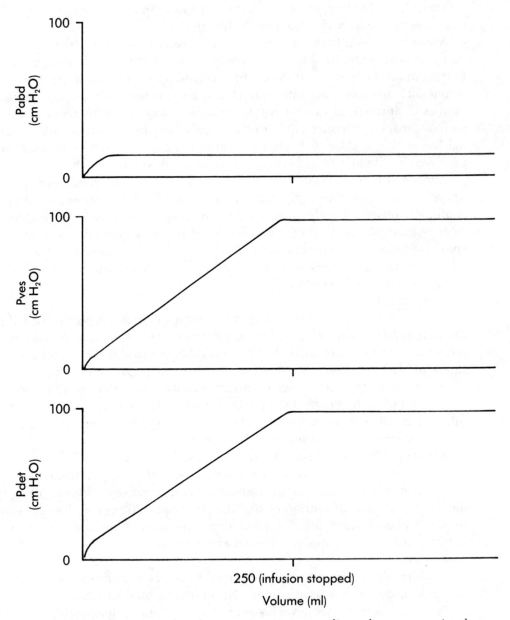

Fig. 3-13 Filling CMG that demonstrates poor compliance by pressure rise that corresponds with increasing volume. Pressure remains elevated despite cessation of infusion, unlike pressure rise followed by decline in pressure, which indicates an unstable detrusor (Fig. 3-14).

of the line showing detrusor pressure that is generated during the normal CMG remains nearly flat (Fig. 3-12).

Compromised compliance is seen as a steady increase in the slope of the detrusor pressure line proportional to volume (Fig. 3-13). Poor bladder wall compliance places the patient at greater risk for infection, upper tract dilatation, vesicoureteral reflux, and compromised renal function.[11,12]

STABILITY

Bladder instability occurs when contractions of the detrusor muscle are not under volitional control.[1] An unstable contraction is seen on the CMG as a spontaneous rise in intravesical *and* detrusor pressure indicating muscle contraction, followed by a decline in pressure associated with muscle relaxation (Fig. 3-14). These contractions are associated with urinary leakage and compromised capacity. They may also produce sensations of urgency. Unstable contractions may be caused by or associated with neurologic disease involving the brain and suprasacral spinal cord segments, stress urinary incontinence, bladder outlet obstruction, irritative disorders, and idiopathic causes.

Sphincter Electromyogram. The filling CMG is accompanied by an EMG of the pelvic floor muscles, or *sphincter EMG*. Sphincter EMG is performed by placing patches over the anal sphincter or by placing needles or hooked wire electrodes into the periurethral muscles. The polygraph recorder then detects electric signals from the periurethral muscles, and a pen sweeps back and forth as electric impulses occur: the wider the sweep of the pen, the greater the muscle tone.

The sphincter response to bladder filling is characterized by a phenomenon called recruitment. Muscle recruitment occurs as the bladder fills; motor units of sphincter muscles are added in response to a greater work load. As a result of recruitment, the EMG sweeps more vigorously as the bladder approaches capacity (Fig. 3-15).

A BCR may be elicited during normal bladder filling and storage. It is produced in women by tapping the clitoris, in men by gently squeezing the glans penis, or by placing light traction against a Foley catheter balloon during filling. A positive BCR is seen as a surge in EMG activity that lasts for several seconds and indicates a grossly intact reflex pathway between sensory receptors of the urethrovesical unit and pelvic floor muscles (Fig. 3-15).

Absence of both the BCR and sphincter recruitment during bladder filling may indicate denervation of these structures. Nonetheless, because of the possibility of artifacts in these measurements, these findings are interpreted within the context of findings from the patient's history and physical examination.

Pressure-Flow Analysis. Urodynamic evaluation of micturition includes a pressure-flow analysis. Pressure-flow analysis is performed after the filling cystom-

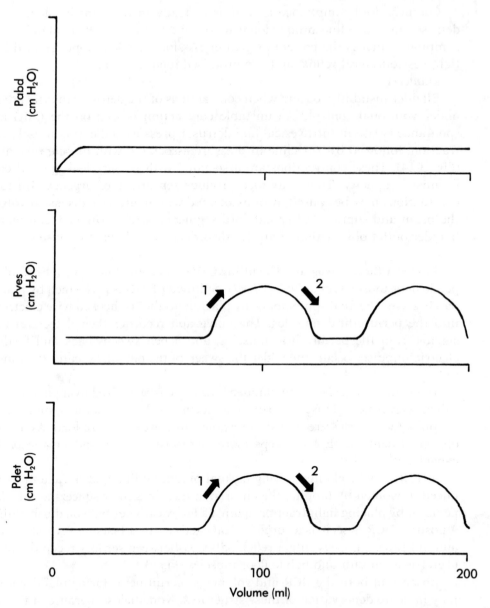

Fig. 3-14   Filling CMG of unstable detrusor. Pressure rise indicates muscle contraction, *1*, followed by a decline in pressure that indicates muscle relaxation, *2*. Pressure rise is seen in *Pves* and *Pdet* channels only.

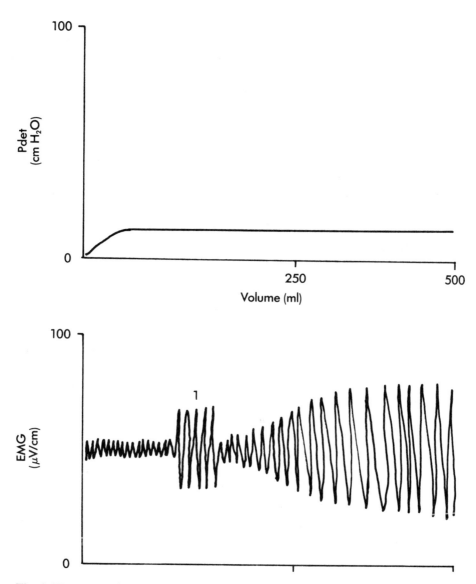

Fig. 3-15 Normal EMG of pelvic floor muscles. Recruitment in response to bladder filling is evident, as is presence of BCR, *1*.

etry. The filling catheter is removed, and a uroflowmeter is used to measure the flow of urine as the patient voids. Fluoroscopy may be performed during this phase of urodynamic evaluation.

The pressure-flow study combines data from the CMG, sphincter EMG, and uroflowmetry to provide a detailed analysis of micturition events. Results of each of these three tests are synthesized with reference to the relationships among contraction pressure, flow, and sphincter response. Analysis of the pressure-flow relationship is begun by determining the urinary flow pattern, as discussed previously in this chapter.

Normal flow pattern. After the flow pattern has been determined, the examiner determines the detrusor pressure and intravesical pressure by the curves produced on the CMG during micturition. In men the maximum bladder contraction, measured as detrusor pressure, ranges from 30 to 60 cm H_2O, and the flow describes a normal pattern with a Qmax greater than 12 ml/sec and a Qave greater than 8 ml/sec. In women, voiding pressures are usually lower and the corresponding flow measurements are greater.

The examiner completes the initial pressure-flow analysis by determining the sphincter response to micturition. Normally the striated sphincter relaxes to allow passage of urine via the urethra. This is seen on urodynamic tracings as a quieting of the EMG pattern. Schematic pressure-flow studies for a man and a woman are shown in Fig. 3-16.

Explosive flow pattern. An understanding of the relationship between pressure, flow, and sphincter response is essential to the interpretation of abnormal findings. For example, the explosive flow pattern is often associated with particularly low micturition pressure and sphincter relaxation in women with stress urinary incontinence (Fig. 3-17). This pattern probably represents low urethral resistance that allows the bladder to empty itself rapidly even at low pressures. As expected, the maximum contraction pressures rise and the maximum and mean flow values decline following bladder neck suspension.[5]

Poor flow pattern. Pressure-flow analysis of the poor flow pattern often reveals abnormally high or low contraction pressures with appropriate sphincter relaxation (Fig. 3-18). If the contraction pressure is high and the flow pattern is poor, the bladder is producing greater than normal energy despite compromised output (flow). High pressure contraction and poor flow indicate bladder outlet obstruction. Quieting of the sphincter EMG indicates appropriate relaxation of pelvic floor muscles and alerts the examiner to search for another source of obstruction.

In contrast, the poor flow pattern may be accompanied by a low contraction pressure or poorly sustained contraction or both. In this case the poor flow occurs because of deficient detrusor contractility.

Intermittent flow pattern. High voiding pressures associated with an intermittent flow pattern also indicate the presence of bladder outlet obstruction.

Text continued on p. 87.

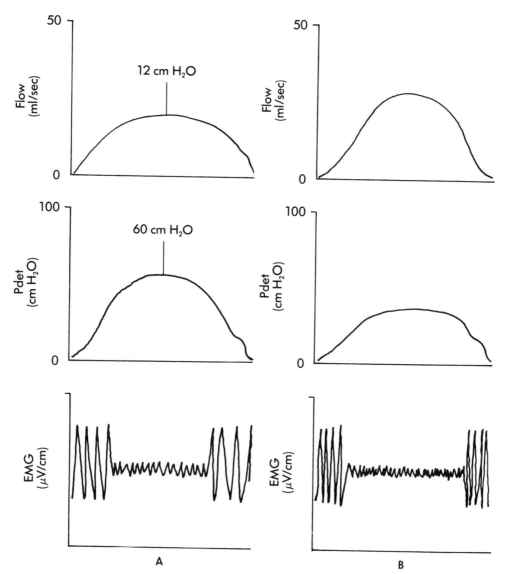

Fig. 3-16   A, Normal pressure-flow analysis of male. **B**, Normal pressure-flow analysis of female.

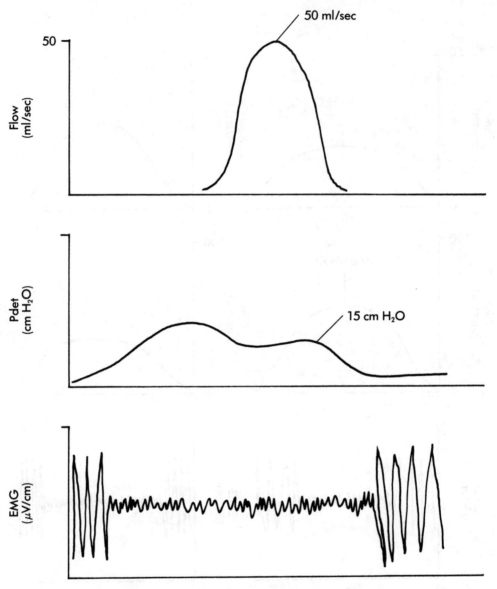

Fig. 3-17   Pressure-flow analysis of woman with stress urinary incontinence showing explosive flow with low pressure contraction and appropriate EMG response.

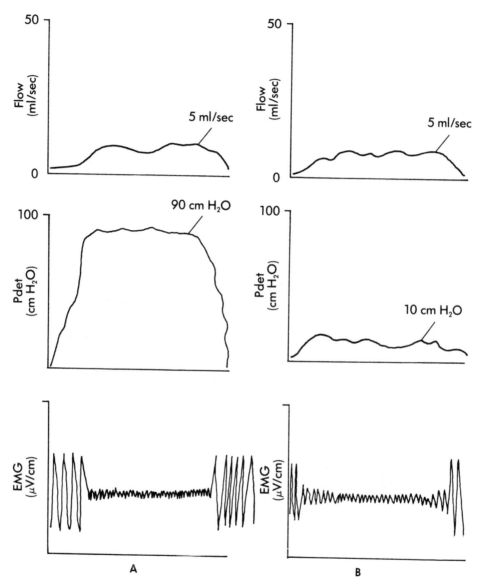

Fig. 3-18 Pressure-flow analysis of poor flow showing, **A**, high pressure with appropriate sphincter response that indicates obstruction and **B**, low pressure contraction with appropriate sphincter response that indicates deficient detrusor contractility.

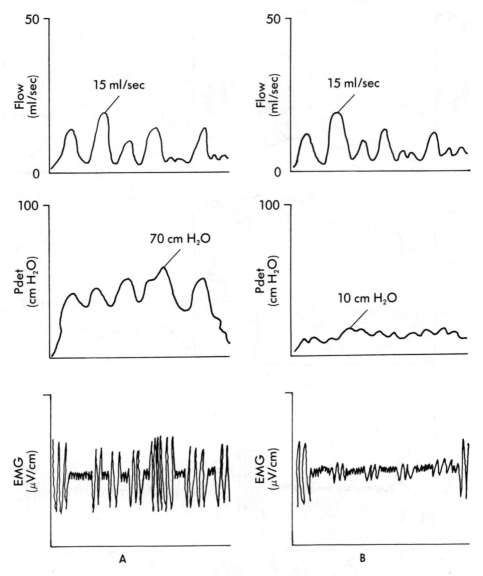

Fig. 3-19   Pressure-flow analysis of intermittent flow demonstrating, **A,** high or adequate pressure contraction and sphincter *dyssynergia* that indicates obstruction at striated sphincter level and, **B,** low pressure contraction with appropriate sphincter response that indicates deficient detrusor contractility.

In certain cases a dyssynergic sphincter may cause dynamic obstruction of the outlet (Fig. 3-19, *A*). The dyssynergic sphincter fails to relax in response to micturition and causes resistance to urinary flow. This condition is seen on the urodynamic tracing as persistent activity during the pressure-flow study.

Intermittent flow pattern associated with low voiding pressures or absent contractions indicates deficient detrusor contractility (Fig. 3-19, *B*). Supplementing a weak detrusor muscle by straining usually produces the intermittency seen in the flow pattern. The urodynamicist observes the abdominal pressure channel of the CMG to document the presence of abdominal enhancement of a poor quality bladder contraction and intermittent flow.

Urethral Pressure Studies. Studies of urethral pressure are used to determine urethral and sphincter behavior during bladder filling and micturition or in response to a specific, stressful event such as a cough. The urethral pressure profile (UPP) is a static test used to determine functional urethral length and maximum urethral closure pressure. Its utility in routine urodynamic assessment remains controversial.[2] Measurement of continuous urethral pressure during bladder filling and evacuation provides dynamic assessment of sphincter function throughout the micturition cycle. Simultaneous measurement of urethral and intravesical pressure during provocative maneuvers such as coughing is used to determine the presence of stress urinary incontinence. Combining urethral pressure measurements with fluoroscopy provides an ideal assessment of sphincter morphology and dynamic pressure responses.[7,16]

PSYCHOSOCIAL CONCERNS
Perceptions and Motivation of Patient

Psychosocial evaluation of the individual with incontinence begins with the health care professional's attempt to gain an understanding of incontinence as it is perceived *through the patient's experience and context of meaning.* This is a surprisingly challenging task because so much of our information about urinary leakage and so many of our preconceived notions about it are derived from our biophysical perspective as health care professionals. Before it is possible to correct or improve the patient's perception of incontinence, it is necessary to determine the meaning of the condition to the patient. This can be ascertained by asking the patient to complete the sentence, "Leaking urine is like . . . "

After gaining an understanding of incontinence from the patient's perspective, the examiner assesses the patient's motivation to engage in a care plan designed to relieve or eliminate the leakage. Again, the examiner must understand the patient's thoughts and feelings before attempting to restructure those perceptions when a particular bladder management program is instituted. The examiner begins by asking the patient to evaluate his or her current bladder management program, including its strengths and weaknesses. This evaluation is particularly valuable after diagnosis, when the examiner is presenting options for management and when altered bladder management strategies are employed.

Perceptions and Concerns of Family and Caregivers

Evaluation of psychosocial concerns related to incontinence includes an assessment of the impact of incontinence on the patient's family or social support structure; incontinence profoundly affects not only the patient's life but also the lives of those close to the patient. For example, incontinence imposes an extra financial burden: the cost of absorptive devices, medications, and related products. The time spent doing laundry may dramatically increase, and family members may resent the patient's reduced ability to participate in social activities. Certainly incontinence also affects sexual relationships.

Ideally the examiner interviews family members or caregivers separately from the patient to encourage frank disclosure of feelings and perceptions. The interview is begun by asking the individual to complete the sentence, "Incontinence in (name of the patient) is like . . . " Again, it is important for the examiner to listen to the family member or caregiver before expressing any judgment or interjecting opinions concerning other ways to view urinary incontinence. In designing a bladder management program the family's motivation for seeking alternative bladder management programs must be considered along with the patient's goals and motivation.

ECONOMIC CONCERNS

It is important to assess the patient and family's economic status and concerns before developing a bladder management program. Management options are limited for some individuals by limited economic resources or health insurance benefits. The nurse often works with a social worker, the patient, and family members to determine what insurance benefits and personal financial resources are available for incontinence management.

SUMMARY

The goals in assessment of the individual with incontinence are to establish an accurate diagnosis, determine the potential for coexisting neurologic or urologic disease, and establish an appropriate bladder management program. The patient history provides clues to the causes of incontinence and current strategies of bladder management. This information is correlated with a limited physical examination of the genitourinary, neurologic, and integumentary systems. Physical examination, laboratory studies, and imaging studies are used to determine the presence of coexisting neurologic or urologic disease or both. Determination of the appropriate bladder management program depends on a comprehensive assessment of the individual's functional capabilities, mentation, environment, psychosocial status, and economic resources. The nurse is uniquely qualified to synthesize these varied data into a physiologically effective, economically sensible, and psychosocially satisfying bladder management program designed to minimize or ablate the consequences of urinary leakage.

SELF-EVALUATION

QUESTIONS

1. Define the following terms and explain the significance of each in the assessment of a patient with urinary incontinence:
   a. Diurnal voiding patterns
   b. Nocturia
   c. Bladder management program

2. Differentiate the following types of incontinence by patient symptoms and patterns of leakage:
   a. Stress incontinence
   b. Instability incontinence
   c. Overflow or paradoxical incontinence
   d. Continuous incontinence
   e. Functional incontinence

3. a. Describe the normal urinary stream.
   b. Explain the significance of an explosive stream, a poor stream, and an intermittent stream.

4. Identify systems to be included in a focused review of systems.

5. Define bulbocavernosus response (BCR) and explain its significance in the assessment of a patient with urinary incontinence.

6. Identify at least three factors to be included in an environmental assessment for the patient with urinary incontinence.

7. Identify key data recorded in a voiding diary.

8. Assessment of a voiding diary should include which of the following data:
   a. Diurnal and nocturnal voiding patterns; usual voiding frequency
   b. Patterns of urinary incontinence
   c. Functional bladder capacity
   d. All of the above

9. List the laboratory and imaging studies that are commonly indicated in the workup of a patient with urinary incontinence.

10. Every patient with urinary incontinence requires complex urodynamic assessment.
    a. True
    b. False

11. Uroflowmetry is frequently performed before cystometrics. Normal results of uroflowmetry indicate:
    a. Effective bladder storage and emptying; no further testing needed
    b. Effective bladder storage; cannot rule out problems with bladder emptying

    c. Effective bladder emptying; cannot rule out problems with bladder storage

    d. None of the above

12. Cystometrogram (CMG) provides assessment of:

    a. Bladder's ability to fill and store

    b. Bladder's ability to empty effectively

    c. Urethral sphincter function

    d. All of the above

13. Identify the four measurements used to assess the bladder's ability to fill and store urine.

14. Sphincter function is assessed by which of the following:

    a. Uroflowmetry

    b. Sphincter electromyogram (EMG)

    c. CMG

    d. IVP

15. Identify the principal assessments included in a pressure-flow analysis.

16. Identify at least three areas to be included in the psychosocial assessment of the patient with urinary incontinence.

17. Which of the following patients requires *immediate* referral for further workup?

    a. Patient with stress incontinence; no residual volume; no evidence of urinary tract infection

    b. Patient with instability (reflex) incontinence; 50% residual volume; symptoms of urinary tract infection

    c. Patient with urge incontinence; low residual volumes; frequency and urgency but negative urinalysis

    d. Patient with constant incontinence related to vesicovaginal fistula caused by terminal cervical cancer

SELF-EVALUATION

ANSWERS

1. **a.** Diurnal voiding patterns: frequency of urination during waking hours. Normal frequency is once every 2 to 6 hours. Excessive frequency indicates sensory urgency disorder, bladder instability, or urinary retention.

   b. Nocturia: condition that occurs when an individual is waked from sleep by the urge to void. Normal frequency is one to two times per night. Greater frequency indicates voiding disorder.

   c. Bladder management program: strategies used by an individual to manage urinary elimination. Common strategies are spontaneous voiding, use of containment devices, indwelling catheter, and intermittent catheterization.

2. **a.** Stress incontinence: urinary leakage produced by physical exertion (such as coughing or sneezing). Not associated with urgency to void. Ranges from mild to severe.

   b. Instability incontinence: contraction of the bladder without its owner's permission. Commonly associated with frequency, urgency, nocturia, and urge incontinence (incontinent episodes preceded by strong urge to void; the patient is unable to delay voiding long enough to reach toilet). In a patient with sensory loss (for example, a patient with a spinal cord injury), instability incontinence may present as reflex incontinence (involuntary voiding triggered by a certain bladder volume or other stimuli; the patient lacks voluntary bladder control or inhibition).

   c. Overflow or paradoxical incontinence: leakage of urine caused by inability to effectively empty the bladder (retention). Signs and symptoms include distention, high residual volumes, frequency, and nocturia.

   d. Continuous incontinence: Incontinence resulting from a congenital or acquired defect that permits urine to bypass normal sphincter mechanism (for example, fistula). Signs and symptoms include constant leakage.

   e. Functional incontinence: incontinence caused by environmental or motivational factors rather than pathologic conditions of the urinary tract or its neural pathways.

3. **a.** Normal stream: begins within 15 seconds of attempt to void; urine is expressed continuously without straining; patient feels that bladder is empty.

   b. Explosive stream: forceful and brief; patient does not strain; may be associated with stress incontinence or may be variant of normal in women. Intermittent stream: requires straining; frequently associated with incomplete emptying and postvoid dribbling. May indicate bladder outlet obstruction or poor bladder contractility. Poor stream: decreased force of stream; may require straining. Frequently associated with post-void dribbling. May be caused by bladder outlet obstruction or poor bladder contractility.

4. Neurologic, genitourinary, gastrointestinal, and integumentary systems
5. Examiner places one gloved, lubricated finger in patient's anus; uses other hand to tap clitoris or squeeze glans penis. Positive BCR occurs when this stimulus produces anal contraction. Positive BCR indicates a grossly intact neural pathway between the pelvic floor muscles and the sacral spinal cord.
6. **a.** Availability of toileting facilities (distance of the bathroom from the living and sleeping areas)
   b. Accessibility of toileting facilities for the patient with assistive devices (wheelchair, walker, and the like)
   c. Safety issues (such as rugs on the floor, slick flooring, dim lighting)
   d. Availability of support bars or handles in the bathroom
7. **a.** Documentation of spontaneous voiding (time and amount)
   b. Documentation of incontinent episodes (time)
   c. Fluid intake patterns (optional)
   d. Activities or circumstances associated with leakage (optional)
8. **d.** All of the above
9. Urinalysis; urine culture and sensitivity; determination of BUN levels and creatinine levels; IVP; ultrasonography
10. False.
11. **c.** Effective bladder emptying; cannot rule out problems with bladder storage
12. **a.** Bladder's ability to fill and store urine
13. Capacity, compliance, sensation, and stability
14. **b.** Sphincter EMG
15. Urinary flow patterns, curves of detrusor pressure and intravesical pressure produced on CMG during micturition, and sphincter response to micturition
16. The concerns and feelings of the patient and family members; the goals of the patient and family members for incontinence management; the patient and family members' understandings of options for management; economic resources; sexual issues
17. **b.** Patient with stress incontinence; 50% residual volume; symptoms of urinary tract infection

REFERENCES

1. Abrams PH: Bladder instability: concept, clinical associations and treatment, Scand J Urol Nephrol 87 [Suppl]:7, 1984.
2. Abrams PH: The urethral pressure profile measurement. In Mundy AR, Stephenson TP, and Wein AJ, eds: Urodynamics: principles, practice, and application, London, 1984, Churchill Livingstone, Inc.
3. Alfaro R: Applying nursing diagnosis and nursing process: a step-by-step guide, ed 2, Philadelphia, 1990, JB Lippincott Co.
4. Clay EC: Incontinence of urine. II and III. Nurs Mirror 146 [10]:36 and [11]:23, 1978.
5. Constantinou CE: Impact of surgery on detrusor contraction strength and pressure/flow parameters, J Neurourol Urodyn 8 [4], [abstract], 1989.
6. Fine EJ and Blaufox MD: Urological applications of radionuclides. In Pollack HM, Clinical urography, vol 1, Philadelphia, 1990, WB Saunders Co.
7. Gray ML: Assessment and investigation of urinary incontinence. In Jeter K, Faller N, and Norton C, eds: Nursing for continence, Philadelphia, 1990, WB Saunders Co.
8. Gray ML: Urinary retention. In Thompson JM et al, eds: Clinical nursing, ed 2, St Louis, 1989, Mosby−Year Book, Inc.
9. Gray ML and Broadwell DC: Genitourinary system. In Thompson JM et al, eds: Clinical nursing, ed 2, St Louis, 1989, Mosby−Year Book, Inc.
10. Gray ML and Dougherty MC: Urinary incontinence: pathophysiology and treatment, J Enterost Ther 14[4]: 152, 1987.
11. Gray ML and Walther MM: Incidental finding of reflux during urodynamics. Paper presented at the Southeastern Section meeting of the American Urological Association, Boca Raton, Fla, March, 1987.
12. Hackler RH and Zampieri TA: Low compliant bladders in the spinal cord injured population, J Urol 139[abstract], 1988.
13. Hirsch JE et al: Dysreflexia. In Thompson JM et al, eds: Clinical nursing, ed 2, St Louis, 1989, Mosby−Year Book, Inc.
14. Norton C: Nursing for continence, Bucks, England, 1986, Beaconsfield Publishers Ltd.
15. Seidel HM et al: Mosby's guide to physical examination, St Louis, 1987, Mosby−Year Book, Inc.
16. Stephenson TP: Dynamic urethral pressure measurements. In Mundy AR, Stephenson TP, and Wein AJ, eds: Urodynamics: principles, practice, and application, London, 1984, Churchill Livingstone, Inc.
17. Tilkian SM, Conover MB, and Tilkian AG: Clinical implications of laboratory tests, St Louis, 1987, Mosby−Year Book, Inc.

4 Management of Urinary Incontinence

MIKEL GRAY
STEVEN W. SIEGEL
RICHARD TROY
NANCY FALLER
ALAN BAKST
BARBARA HOCEVAR

OBJECTIVES

1. Identify treatments and considerations for each of the following:
   Patient with stress incontinence
   Patient with instability (urge) incontinence
   Patient with instability (reflex) incontinence
   Patient with overflow incontinence
   Patient with continual (total) incontinence
   Patient with functional aspects that contribute to incontinence

2. Identify indications for surgical intervention in the management of urinary incontinence.

3. Explain the goal in the surgical management of stress incontinence caused by:
   Pelvic floor relaxation and bladder neck displacement
   Intrinsic sphincter dysfunction

4. Identify patients who are candidates for the artificial urinary sphincter (AUS).

5. Describe the three parts of the AUS in terms of location, function, and operation.

6. Explain how bladder augmentation contributes to management of patients with instability incontinence.

7. Describe the following medications in terms of mechanism of action and indications for use in the management of urinary incontinence:
   Anticholinergic or smooth-muscle relaxant drugs
   Alpha-adrenergic agonists
   Cholinergic drugs
   Alpha-adrenergic blocking agents

8. Identify patients who may benefit from a program of clean intermittent catheterization.

9. Describe the main points in a teaching program for the patient who is beginning clean intermittent catheterization.

10. Identify patients who may benefit from a program of pelvic floor exercises.

11. Describe two ways to teach the patient to isolate the periurethral muscles.

12. Identify patients who are likely to respond to toileting programs.

13. Differentiate a program of prompted voiding from a bladder drill program in terms of program goals, instructions to the patient, and necessary levels of support for the patient.

14. Identify situations in which an indwelling catheter is the treatment of choice for the management of urinary incontinence.

15. Develop a care plan for the patient with an indwelling catheter, including the following: the type and size of catheter to be used; indications for change; routine care of catheter, periurethral area, and drainage system; indications for urine culture; and management of leakage.

16. Describe options for urine containment for patients with intractable incontinence.

17. Explain appropriate skin care for patients who are using containment devices, including routine cleansing, the correct use of protective products, and the management of skin breakdown.

18. Identify the two factors thought to contribute to enuresis and the treatment options associated with each factor.

19. Identify the two goals for the management of patients with urinary incontinence.

INTERVENTIONS FOR RESTORATION OF CONTINENCE

Two principal objectives direct nursing care for patients with urinary incontinence. To prevent or ablate urinary leakage is the first goal of care whenever feasible; when a cure is not attainable, urinary containment with proper skin care becomes the objective. A second, equally important objective of care for the incontinent patient is to prevent or minimize any deterioration in renal function so that the patient's health is maintained.

Interventions for Patients with Stress Incontinence

The pathophysiology of stress urinary incontinence involves alterations in urethrovesical anatomy (pelvic floor relaxation) or reduced competence of the sphincter mechanism or both. Interventions to alleviate or cure stress incontinence promote urethral closure (increased competence of the sphincter mechanism) or reestablish more normal urethrovesical anatomy. Treatment options include pelvic floor exercises, pharmacologic manipulation, pessary devices, and surgical procedures designed to restore normal urethrovesical anatomy or to support urethral competence.

Pelvic Floor Exercises. Pelvic floor exercises are based on principles of exercise physiology; the individual with incontinence is taught to strengthen the striated muscle component of the sphincter mechanism. The potential benefits of pelvic floor exercises in the treatment of stress urinary incontinence were first described by Kegel.[29] Since that time, Kegel's exercises have been prescribed for women to help restore pelvic floor strength in the postpartum period[9] or to regain urinary control in cases of mild to moderate stress urinary incontinence.

The success of pelvic floor physiotherapy depends on proper instruction and supervision by a health care professional; the goals are to ensure that patients perform the exercises accurately and to promote adherence to a regular exercise program, sometimes for several weeks or months, until results are evident.[24]

Commercially produced pelvic floor exercise systems that are also based on principles of exercise physiology are now available. These systems operate from a central computer in the office or clinic; units that patients take home record and store data when patients exercise outside the office or clinic. These systems are useful for exercise instruction because they provide noninvasive, reliable feedback about the compliance of patients and the effectiveness of home exercise regimens.

Isolation of periurethral muscles. The patient is first taught to isolate and contract the periurethral muscles. When patients first attempt to exercise the pelvic floor, they often have difficulty isolating and contracting the proper muscle. Typically the abdominal or thigh muscles are exercised while the periurethral muscles remain unused.

Several methods may be used to help the patient identify and work the proper muscles during Kegel exercises. Dougherty et al.[8,9] used an assessment system consisting of the following devices: a strip chart recorder, a custom-designed intravaginal balloon that is used to evaluate the efficiency and magnitude of circumvaginal muscle contraction, and a posterior vaginal balloon that is used to assess abdominal pressure. Using a two-channel strip chart recorder, Dougherty et al. were able to distinguish the contraction of circumvaginal (periurethral) muscles from the contraction of abdominal muscles. This system serves a dual purpose: it allows evaluation of preexercise strength and endurance of the circumvaginal muscle, and it provides feedback that helps a woman identify and contract the appropriate muscles.

Other strategies can be devised to help individuals identify the periurethral muscles. Contraction of the pelvic floor muscles may be assessed by using percutaneous wire electrodes, needles, or patches. Patch electrodes placed at the anal sphincter reflect contraction of the periurethral muscles; a simultaneous recording of abdominal muscle activity by electromyography provides feedback regarding inadvertent contraction of these muscles.

Simple methods may also be used to help patients identify the periurethral muscles. The nurse may gently place a gloved finger in the anterior vaginal vault (in women) or the distal anal canal (in men). The appropriate muscle group is described to the patient, and he or she is asked to contract the muscle while the nurse's gloved finger remains in the vagina or anus. Contraction of the pelvic floor muscles causes apposition of the posterior and anterior vaginal walls (in women) or circumferential contraction of the anal sphincter (in men). The nurse determines contraction of inappropriate muscle groups by simultaneously placing the free hand on the patient's abdomen or buttocks. The nurse repeats the maneuver until the patient consistently isolates and contracts the pelvic floor muscles while abdominal and thigh muscles remain relaxed.

The nurse reassures the patient that several of these sessions are usually necessary before patients can expect to consistently contract the pelvic floor muscles without inadvertently tightening other muscle groups. Training sessions should be scheduled for a time when the patient is not fatigued or preoccupied. The patient is asked to contract the pelvic floor muscles several times and in different positions to identify which position gives best results. The nurse uses follow-up and evaluation sessions to reinforce teaching; when expected improvements do not occur, the nurse must repeat the initial instructions.

Home exercise program. After teaching the patient to correctly contract the pelvic floor muscles, the nurse provides the patient with written and verbal instructions for a home exercise regimen. The regimen consists of two types of exercises, exercises for strength and exercises for endurance. The individual is taught to increase strength by contracting the periurethral muscles as tightly as possible for 6 seconds while maintaining the gluteal and abdominal muscles in a relaxed state. This exercise is repeated 15 times with 10-second rest periods between contractions. The patient is begun on a regimen of 15 repetitions 3 days per week and advanced in increments of 2 repetitions per week to a maximum of 25 repetitions 3 days per week.[9]

The patient is taught to improve endurance by contracting the periurethral muscles and maintaining the contraction for 12 seconds. Initially the patient is instructed to hold the contraction for 6 seconds; the contraction period is increased by 2 seconds per week until the patient can hold each contraction for 12 seconds. A maximum of 30 repetitions 3 days per week is recommended by Dougherty.[9] Other clinicians may recommend slightly different schedules.

Evaluation of effectiveness. The success of a pelvic floor exercise program may be evaluated (1) by subjective reports provided by the patient, (2) by perineometry of the periurethral muscles, (3) by a pad test that quantifies the volume of leakage, or (4) by complex urodynamics. Subjective reports are discouraged, since patients are quick to report improvement even when objective measurements show little or no improvement, perhaps because they are anxious to please a clinician who has shown an interest in this often ignored problem. Perineometry offers the advantage of direct and objective assessment of the efficiency of muscle contraction. Although pad testing and complex urodynamics may yield less encouraging findings than perineometry,[24] they offer a more direct assessment of the *desired result* of pelvic floor exercises (that is, reduction in stress incontinence) rather than an evaluation of muscle strength and endurance.

Pessary Devices. Stress incontinence in women may also be managed by placement of an appropriate pessary device. A pessary device is a ring-shaped, doughnut-shaped, spherical, or oblong device manufactured of vulcanized rubber or some inert material. After a physician (gynecologist) has been consulted, the device is placed in the vaginal vault and replaced as necessary.[56]

The pessary relieves symptoms of stress incontinence by mechanically restoring a more normal urethrovesical position. It promotes more effective urethral closure by relocating the sphincter mechanism to the optimal position for effective closure. A pessary may be used for those women with significant pelvic floor relaxation and uterine prolapse who are not candidates for (or do not benefit from) exercise regimens and who are not candidates for surgery.

The success of pessary placement depends on proper insertion by an experienced physician or nurse specialist. Follow-up care is essential; the patient must be monitored for adverse reactions, including vaginal erosion and adherence of the device to the vaginal walls.[56] Pessaries are further discussed later in this chapter in the section on the management of intractable incontinence.

Pharmacologic Manipulation. Stress incontinence may also respond to pharmacologic manipulation. Women with evidence of estrogen deficiency may be treated with topical or systemic estrogens. Alpha-adrenergic (sympathomimetic) drugs may also help to alleviate stress incontinence. Sympathomimetics are available as over-the-counter (nonprescription) medications; however, they should be taken according to a physician's direction. The patient is directed to take preparations that contain an alpha-sympathomimetic drug *without* caffeine or histamine (such as ephedrine, pseudoephedrine, or phenylpropanolamine). The nurse's role is to teach the patient how and when to take these medications and how to monitor for side effects. The nurse explains that these drugs are marketed as diet pills or decongestants but that they also help to increase urethral resistance and thus are beneficial in the management of stress incontinence. The patient is instructed to take the medication only during waking hours, since stress incontinence is rarely a problem during sleep and since these preparations can cause insomnia. Side effects of alpha-sympathomimetic drugs include anxiety, insomnia, and palpitations.[21] Proper scheduling and dosage of medication may alleviate these symptoms; patients are instructed to contact the nurse or physician should problems occur. Alpha-sympathomimetic drugs are used with caution in patients with hypertension: a regular schedule is established for monitoring blood pressure, and the patient is instructed to discontinue the drug and contact the physician promptly should his or her blood pressure rise above desired levels.

Stress incontinence complicated by urge (instability) incontinence may be treated with imipramine, which relieves the symptoms of bladder instability (urgency, frequency, urge incontinence, and nocturia), and exerts a mild alpha-adrenergic effect to promote urethral closure. Common side effects of imipramine are dry mouth, constipation, and urinary retention. Nursing implications for the use of imipramine and other anticholinergic agents are addressed later in this chapter in the discussion of the management of instability incontinence. Pharmacologic intervention is discussed on pp. 125-128. Surgical options for management of stress incontinence are discussed on pp. 112-121.

Intervention for Patients with Instability Incontinence

Instability incontinence occurs when the smooth muscle of the bladder wall (detrusor) contracts "without its owner's permission," causing urinary leakage. When sensations of urgency and fullness in the lower urinary tract are perceived, the symptom of *urge incontinence* occurs. In contrast, when spinal cord abnormalities cause a loss of lower urinary tract sensations, *reflex incontinence* results.

Urge Incontinence. The goal in managing urge incontinence is to reduce bladder instability and improve the patient's bladder control. Treatment options include elimination of any bladder irritants, prompted voiding or bladder drill programs, pharmacologic manipulation, electrostimulation, and biofeedback therapy.

Elimination of bladder irritants. As discussed in Chapter 3, bladder irritants such as infection rarely cause incontinence; however, irritant factors can exacerbate urinary frequency and leakage and should be eliminated. Common irritants include lower urinary tract infections, bladder calculi, caffeinated or citrus beverages, and some bath preparations (for example, bubble baths). The patient should be assessed for evidence of such irritants, and appropriate measures should be taken to eliminate them.

Prompted voiding and bladder drill programs. Patients with urge incontinence are initially managed by prompted voiding or bladder drill regimens. A prompted voiding program consists of asking the patient to void "by the clock." The individual is placed on a schedule that is determined by the functional capacity and frequency data from the patient's voiding diary. (Voiding is usually scheduled to occur at 1½-hour intervals during the day.) The goals of a prompted voiding program are to determine how long the patient can realistically postpone voiding and to teach the individual to void volitionally before leakage occurs.

Bladder drill therapy is similar to a prompted voiding regimen in that the patient is asked to void according to a timed schedule. Unlike the prompted voiding schedule, however, bladder drill regimens help the patient to *increase* functional capacity by using behavioral techniques. The patient is begun on a voiding schedule of 1½-hour intervals, and he or she is instructed to adhere strictly to the regimen despite feelings of urgency or occurrence of leakage. The schedule is discontinued at night. As the patient becomes proficient at this interval (able to remain consistently dry), the interval is increased in half-hour increments to 2 hours and so on until the patient is voiding every 3 or 4 hours.

The success of a bladder drill regimen depends on persistent and intensive nursing support and supervision. The nurse explains the procedure and its goals to the patient and establishes an initial contract in which the patient agrees to continue therapy for some realistic period of time (at least 2 to 4 weeks) to allow an adequate trial phase. During therapy, the patient is contacted frequently. The nurse provides opportunities for the individual to express difficulties encountered in adhering to the drill and encourages continuing subjective evaluation of results. When regimens are followed, bladder drill therapy is reported to be even more effective than pharmacologic therapy among women with idiopathic instability.[16,27] Its role in the management of patients with neuropathic instability involving diseases of the brain remains to be elucidated.

Fluid control. Bladder drill or prompted voiding regimens are complemented by programs to control fluid intake. The goal of a fluid control regimen is to distribute the intake of beverages throughout waking hours, so that the incontinent urinary system is not forced to cope with a large volume of liquid in a brief period of time. The patient is advised to maintain a fluid intake of at least 1000 to 2500 ml per day, to abstain from drinking large quantities of fluids with meals (usually no more than 8 ounces), to sip liquids between meals, and to discontinue fluid consumption approximately 2 hours before sleep to alleviate nocturia.

Pharmacologic manipulation. Patients who do not respond to bladder drill or prompted voiding regimens because of markedly reduced functional bladder capacity are managed by antispasmodic or anticholinergic medications prescribed by a physician. The goal of pharmacologic therapy is to increase functional bladder capacity by decreasing detrusor contractility; drugs may be used alone or in combination (for example, propantheline, oxybutinin, flavoxate, or imipramine). The nurse teaches the individual the proper dosage and schedule for the drug, and teaches him or her to recognize and manage side effects. The nurse also reminds the patient that antispasmodic medications are most effective when they are used as a *portion* of a bladder management program that includes prompted voiding and fluid control.

Occasionally, pharmacologic agents are used to paralyze the bladder. In this case the goal of therapy is to administer enough antispasmodic medication to ablate all unstable contractions; intermittent catheterization is then employed to ensure regular, complete bladder evacuation. Pharmacologic paralysis is most advantageous when urge incontinence is complicated by significant urinary retention, particularly when detrusor contractility is deficient. Nonetheless, pharmacologic paralysis with intermittent catheterization has only limited use in the management of patients with urge incontinence. Side effects of the drug, adjustment to an intermittent catheterization program by an individual accustomed to spontaneous voiding, discomfort associated with initial attempts at catheterization, and the risk of breakthrough contractions with leakage significantly limit patient acceptance of this strategy.

Nursing management of incontinence in patients who are taking antispasmodic medications and employing clean intermittent catheterization centers on teaching patients correct technique for catheterization and the proper dosage and scheduling of antispasmodic medications. Identification and management of side effects caused by antispasmodic medications (dry mouth and constipation)[21] is emphasized because particularly large doses are required to paralyze the unstable detrusor. Instruction in clean intermittent catheterization is discussed on pp. 103-105.

Electrostimulation and biofeedback therapy. Other strategies less commonly used in the United States in the management of urge incontinence include electrostimulation and biofeedback therapy. Electrostimulation, performed by placing a probe in the rectum or vagina, causes inhibition of the pelvic plexus with ablation of unstable detrusor contractions.[37] Electrostimulation therapy sessions are performed in the clinic or at home; sessions generally last 20 minutes and are repeated as often as once every 1 to 4 days. Electrostimulation therapy resulted in an initial cure rate of approximately 50% when objective and subjective criteria were used; approximately 77% of patients remained symptom free for 1 year after completion of therapy.[13]

Biofeedback therapy has also been employed in the management of bladder instability and urge incontinence: the patient is taught to suppress unstable contractions by contracting the pelvic floor muscles. Although results of short-term biofeedback therapy have been encouraging, follow-up studies have demonstrated a significant rate of recurrence.[6]

Reflex Incontinence. The goal in the management of the patient with reflex incontinence is to establish a program that provides the patient with a socially acceptable level of urinary dryness while protecting the kidneys from damage.

Because reflex incontinence results from suprasacral spinal cord lesions (lesions above the S2 vertebral level), bladder instability typically coexists with vesico-sphincter dyssynergia. Dyssynergia, or incoordination between the detrusor muscle and the urethral sphincter mechanism, produces a functional obstruction that causes urinary retention. A successful bladder management program for the patient with reflex incontinence and dyssenergia must eliminate or contain urinary leakage while preventing the infection, urinary tract dilatation, and compromised renal function associated with obstruction. Treatment options include clean intermittent catheterization, pharmacologic manipulation, and condom drainage with or without sphincterotomy.

Clean intermittent catheterization. Clean intermittent catheterization is quite often the best bladder management program for patients with reflex incontinence and dyssynergia. Clean intermittent catheterization provides complete, regular bladder emptying and is associated with an acceptably low rate of urinary tract infection, particularly as compared to urethral or suprapubic catheter drainage.[34] A clean intermittent catheterization schedule of 4 times daily during waking hours is considered ideal, although more frequent catheterization may be required. For the patient with reflex incontinence, clean intermittent catheterization may be combined with antispasmodic pharmacotherapy, which ablates unstable contractions and prevents leakage between catheterizations. Antispasmodic medications also prevent unstable, high-pressure bladder contractions that stress the urinary system.

The nurse is responsible for teaching the patient to perform self-catheterization and for providing family members or other caregivers with the skills necessary to assist the patient or perform the procedure. Ideally, teaching begins soon after spinal cord injury or loss of bladder control. Clean intermittent catheterization is initially performed by nursing staff; the patient and other caregivers become independent by their gradually increased involvement in the procedure.

ISSUES RELATED TO PERINEAL ACCESS

The nurse begins instruction in clean intermittent catheterization by assessing issues related to perineal access; this assessment is particularly important for women and girls, who must be able to attain and maintain labial separation. For the patient with normal mobility and dexterity, perineal access is not a problem; he or she may catheterize in a standing or seated position, depending on preference. For the patient with reduced mobility or dexterity or both the nurse must determine the optimal position for catheterization and ascertain the patient's ability to manipulate clothing and adequately expose the urethral meatus for catheter insertion. For example, the patient with paraplegia is usually taught to catheterize from a wheelchair: a man or boy may need to wear clothing with Velcro closures or loose elastic waistbands to successfully expose and instrument the urethra from the sitting position; a woman or girl may need to wear clothing that facilitates perineal exposure, and it may be necessary for her to shift forward and position one leg over the arm of the wheelchair. The patient with quadriplegia may need assistive devices (such as tenodesis splints) or help from another person to catheterize successfully. The elderly patient with arthritis may also find it difficult to manipulate clothing or the catheter or both. An occupational therapist may be consulted to help select appropriate assistive devices. If the patient is unable to achieve positioning and urethral exposure independently and does not have assistance, an alternative bladder management program must be developed.

PRINCIPLES AND PROCEDURE OF PATIENT INSTRUCTION

The nurse begins instruction by explaining the principles of *clean* catheterization. These are simply stated: clean, dry hands and a clean, well-lubricated catheter. The nurse demonstrates and teaches proper handwashing technique and helps the patient identify appropriate alternatives for cleaning the hands when soap and water are not readily available. Initially, the nurse catheterizes the patient while discussing principles and techniques of the procedure. The patient and caregivers are then taught to wash their hands and the patient's urethral meatus, to manipulate and lubricate the catheter, and finally, to insert the catheter and drain the bladder of urine. A mirror may be used during initial attempts to help a woman or girl correctly identify the urethra; the goal, however, is to teach the patient to locate the urethral meatus by palpation.

CATHETER CARE

The nurse also teaches patients to choose and care for their catheters. For women, short, clear catheters are used; clear plastic catheters or red rubber catheters are used for men. In certain instances a coudé-tipped catheter is used to negotiate sharp angles in the urethral course. The individual and caregivers are taught to rinse the catheter with cool water immediately after use to remove sediment and to thoroughly clean the catheter before using it again. They are taught to avoid storing catheters in any type of antiseptic solution. Instead, the catheter is cleaned in warm, soapy water, rinsed well, dried thoroughly, and stored in a dry place. The nurse helps the patient identify and design storage containers for catheters that are appropriate for home use and for use when the patient is away from home. The patient needs containers for both clean and used catheters; these containers should be air permeable and inexpensive. A container used outside the home should be easily concealable in a purse or pocket.

The nurse teaches the individual to clean catheters by one of two methods. (1) The catheter is rinsed with cool water immediately after use and stored in a "dirty" container. Before reuse, the external surface and internal lumen of the catheter must be thoroughly washed with a bacteriostatic soap and water, rinsed well, and allowed to dry thoroughly. The patient is taught *not* to store the catheter in any solution. (2) The catheter is sterilized at home in a microwave oven.[10] Although the indications for home sterilization of catheters remain unestablished, this approach may be useful for the patient who has recurrent urinary tract infections despite a regimen of clean intermittent catheterization. Sterilization includes thorough cleaning and rinsing of the catheters as previously described. Immediately after rinsing, as many as six catheters may be placed in a self-sealing (Ziploc) plastic bag so that moisture is retained. The bag is then placed in a microwave oven and heated for 12 minutes. The patient is advised to check for and avoid cold spots in the microwave (by using a unit with a rotating platform or by using heat-sensitive paper to locate cold spots).

PREVENTION AND MANAGEMENT OF COMPLICATIONS

In addition to teaching the patient the principles and procedure for clean intermittent catheterization and the appropriate care of catheters, the nurse teaches the patient how to monitor for and respond to possible complications associated with his or her bladder dysfunction and bladder management program. Key instructional points include the following:

1. Recognition and management of urethral trauma. The patient is advised to contact his or her physician promptly should any significant bleeding occur with catheterization, or if blood is grossly visible in the urine.
2. Recognition of urinary tract infection. The patient is taught to recognize possible indications of bacteriuria; persistently cloudy, concentrated urine, the presence of blood or sediment in urine, or the recurrence of leakage (instability incontinence). The patient is also taught to recognize the signs of serious infection involving the kidneys: a temperature greater than 100° F, nausea and vomiting, and discomfort in the flank or back. The patient with spinal cord damage is reminded that sensory loss associated with that condition masks the typical symptoms of dysuria and frequency.
3. Management of urinary tract infection. For symptoms of lower urinary tract infection (bacteriuria), the patient is advised to increase the daily oral intake of fluid to 2500 ml immediately, to notify the physician or nurse of probable infection so that a urine culture and sensitivity test may be performed, and to complete any course of antibiotic drugs the physician may prescribe. For symptoms of upper urinary tract infection (febrile illness or the inability to tolerate food or oral fluids) the patient is advised to seek medical attention immediately.
4. Side effects related to anticholinergic medications. Patients who are taking anticholinergic medications to reduce bladder instability are advised of the possible side effects of anticholinergic medications, for example, dry mouth and constipation. The individual is taught to recognize possible indications of drug toxicity (for example, hallucinations or blurred vision) and to discontinue use of the drug and notify the physician promptly should such signs occur.

Reflex voiding and condom drainage. Males whose incontinence cannot be controlled by clean intermittent catheterization and antispasmodic pharmacotherapy, or who cannot catheterize themselves because of physical disability, may manage their bladders with a program of reflex voiding and depend on external catheter (condom) drainage for urine containment. Such a program is feasible only for patients who do not have bladder-sphincter dyssynergia or for patients with dyssynergia that can be controlled by medications or surgical sphincterotomy. Complex urodynamic testing is used to assess the patient for obstructive dyssynergia and to evaluate the long-term safety of a reflex voiding program; alpha-adrenergic blocking agents (for example, prazosin or terazosin) or surgical sphincterotomy may be used to reduce urethral sphincter resistance when indicated. Further reconstructive surgery (for example, continent diversion), may be necessary for the patient with dyssynergia that is not adequately managed by pharmacologic or surgical sphincterotomy.

For the patient who is using a program of reflex voiding for bladder management, nursing management focuses on care of the condom drainage device and prevention of associated complications. An external (condom) catheter that contains urinary leakage without compromising skin integrity of the penis is chosen. The device should provide adequate adherence to the penile shaft and sufficient stiffness at the distal end to prevent twisting and trapping of urine when voiding occurs. If the patient is also using a program of intermittent catheterization, a condom drainage device that does not have to be removed during catheterization should be chosen. The use of external catheters is further discussed on p. 132.

The nurse also helps the patient select an appropriate leg bag for urine collection. The ideal leg bag has a cloth or air-permeable backing to protect the skin, and straps are composed of a material that stretches to hold the leg bag in place despite shearing forces caused by normal movement. The proximal or infusion port of the bag should have an antireflux mechanism, and the distal port should have an outlet that can be manipulated easily by a quadriplegic who has no "pincher" grasp. (The outlet must be secure enough to prevent unintentional drainage, however.) The leg bag should baffle urine so that the bag does not bulge noticeably as it fills.

Key points in instruction for the patient who is managing reflex incontinence with condom drainage include the prevention of skin breakdown and the prevention and management of urinary tract infection. The importance of long-term follow-up care (including a repeat of the urodynamic assessment and imaging studies of the upper urinary tract) is emphasized.

Intervention for Patients with Overflow Incontinence (Urinary Retention)

Urinary retention is caused by deficient detrusor function or bladder outlet obstruction. Overflow incontinence, a dribbling leakage of urine accompanied by an inability to empty the bladder, is a presenting symptom of urinary retention, as are urinary frequency and nocturia. The nursing management of urinary retention and overflow incontinence is directed toward eliminating urinary stasis and correcting or managing incontinence.

After determining the cause of urinary retention, the nurse, in consultation with the urologist, initiates a bladder management program. When urinary retention occurs because of outlet obstruction, the initial management program is designed to promote urinary elimination until surgical correction of the obstruction is completed. If retention occurs because of deficient detrusor function, the program is employed for a longer time. Treatment options may include double voiding and fluid control programs, pharmacologic manipulation, clean intermittent catheterization, indwelling catheter, and surgical correction of the underlying obstruction.

Double Voiding and Fluid Control Programs. A program of double voiding may be effective in cases of mild to moderate outlet obstruction. The patient is taught to void twice during each trip to the bathroom to reduce residual urine volumes. The patient is instructed to void, remain on the toilet, and void again after a rest period of several minutes.

A program of fluid control may also benefit the person with urinary retention. The nurse explains to the patient that adequate fluid intake must be maintained daily but that distributing the intake of fluids throughout waking hours and curtailing intake before sleep may help control symptoms of urinary frequency and nocturia.

Pharmacologic Manipulation. Pharmacologic manipulation may also be used to relieve urinary retention caused by outlet obstruction. Alpha-adrenergic blocking agents such as prazosin or terazosin may be prescribed by the physician to promote proximal urethral funneling during micturition, thus reducing retention. For patients who are receiving alpha-adrenergic blocking agents to relieve urinary frequency, nursing management focuses on teaching the patient the proper dosage and scheduling of the drug and management of side effects. Postural hypotension and dizziness are significant side effects of these agents.[23] Patients should be advised to rise slowly; if dizziness is a problem, patients should be advised to sit and briefly exercise the legs before standing.

For the patient who is managing incomplete emptying with a program of double voiding, fluid control, pharmacologic manipulation, or a combination of these, instruction must include measures for the management of acute urinary retention. Acute urinary retention is recognized by the abrupt cessation of micturition followed by increasing feelings of suprapubic discomfort as the bladder fills without relief. This condition is particularly common in men with prostatic outlet obstruction.[27] The nurse advises the patient to relax, sit in a tub of warm water or stand in a warm shower, and attempt to void. Drinking warm tea may also help stimulate micturition. If these simple procedures fail, the patient is advised to seek help from his or her physician or from an emergency care facility. The nurse also advises the patient with prostatic outlet obstruction to avoid factors that may precipitate an episode of acute urinary retention. Severe chills, consumption of large amounts of alcohol, and the use of over-the-counter cold medicines or diet pills containing alpha-adrenergic agents may all contribute to bladder neck closure and interruption of micturition. The patient should also be advised to consult with his or her physician before taking any prescribed antidepressant or anticholinergic drugs, since these drugs also can precipitate acute retention.[27]

Intermittent Catheterization. Intermittent catheterization may be used to manage urinary retention. Catheterization provides regular, complete bladder evacuation, helps to prevent urinary tract infection, and prevents the deleterious effects of high-pressure voiding in the patient with outlet obstruction. Principles of clean intermittent catheterization are included in the discussion of reflex incontinence.

Indwelling Catheter. An indwelling catheter is sometimes necessary for the management of urinary retention. Ideally, the indwelling catheter is used only until a more definitive management program can be established. Occasionally, long-term catheter drainage is necessary. The nurse selects the type of catheter and drainage system to be used; insertion of a catheter is performed according to the direction of a physician.

Catheter selection. The indwelling urinary catheter should be constructed of a material that minimizes irritation and damage to the urethral mucosa. Traditionally, latex catheters coated with Teflon or Silastic were used; because inflammation was associated with use of latex catheters, inert materials such as silicone gained in popularity. Recently, catheters have been manufactured from hydrogel materials. These materials offer several potential advantages, including greater biocompatibility with the urethral mucosa, reduction of friction and local cell damage, and alleviation of discomfort associated with local inflammation. Although clinical experience has been positive with newer catheter designs, systematic research that compares various catheter materials is necessary.

Catheter selection should also include consideration of drainage capacity. The ratio of external diameter (French size) to internal diameter is important. The nurse should remember that the external size of the catheter does not imply a drainage lumen of equal size. Therefore, the thicker the wall of the catheter, the greater the French size required to provide adequate drainage, particularly in the presence of debris such as blood clots or strands of mucus. Typically a

French size 16 or size 18 catheter is adequate for adults; pediatric catheters range from a French size 8 to size 12, depending on the child's age and size.

Management of drainage system. The patient must also learn to care for a drainage system. The characteristics of an ideal leg bag are discussed in the section on reflex incontinence. The individual with an indwelling catheter also needs an effective system for drainage at night. The reservoir should be large enough to store the urinary output for an 8-hour period (at least 2 liters). The drainage system should have tubing that can be attached to a bedside rail or some supportive device beside the bed, and it should have a drainage port that is easily manipulated but remains closed during movement. The tubing should be long enough to reach a resting spot below the patient's bladder but short enough to prevent the twisting that impedes drainage. The patient is taught how to drain and rinse the drainage system and to routinely clean the system. A solution of hydrogen peroxide or vinegar can be used to reduce the growth of bacteria and associated odor.

For the patient with an indwelling catheter the nurse emphasizes the importance of maintenance care and routine follow-up: adequate daily fluid intake; indications for routine catheter change; recognition of signs of urinary tract infection (suprapubic discomfort or flank discomfort, fever, or cloudy, malodorous urine); prompt treatment for symptomatic infections; routine medical reevaluation; and medical evaluation as necessary for problems associated with the catheter (for example, leakage or discomfort).[46]

Intervention for Patients with Continual Incontinence

Continual (extraurethral or constant) incontinence most commonly results from congenital anomalies or disease processes that affect the structure of the urinary system and bypass the urethral sphincter mechanism (for example, ectopic ureters or fistulas involving the bladder): the result is uncontrolled leakage of urine. Treatment options include surgical correction of the structural anomaly, use of containment devices and skin protection, and urinary diversion. The use of containment devices and skin protection is discussed on pp. 135-138, and urinary diversion is discussed on p. 122.

Intervention for Patients with Functional Incontinence

Functional incontinence is a nursing diagnosis that implies loss of bladder control related to a functional deficit rather than to organic dysfunction.[22,30] In clinical practice, functional incontinence is relatively exotic as an isolated finding. More commonly, the four types of incontinence (stress, instability, overflow, and continuous) are complicated or exacerbated by functional deficits; a comprehensive, effective nursing management plan must include measures to alleviate the functional aspects of urinary leakage, as well as strategies to treat the voiding dysfunction itself.

Functional deficits that contribute to incontinence can be classified into three broad categories. Deficits of mobility or access include physiological or environmental factors that limit the patient's mobility or access to toilet facilities as needed. Deficits related to dexterity affect continence by limiting the individual's ability to manipulate clothing before voiding. Deficits in *mentation* affect continence when the person cannot process and synthesize either the environmental and sensory indicators of the need to empty the bladder or the steps necessary to complete this task.

Mobility and Access Deficits. Limited mobility is a common finding in patients with urinary incontinence. Persons with neuropathic bladder dysfunction may be confined to a wheelchair or may ambulate only with assistive devices such as braces or a walker. The elderly person's mobility may be limited by arthritis or impaired sight. Nursing intervention for these individuals focuses on increasing their mobility and access to toilet facilities.

The patient with limited mobility is helped to obtain appropriate assistive devices such as a cane, braces, a wheelchair, or a walker. The nurse evaluates the patient's shoes and encourages the patient to switch from slick-heeled slippers to nonskid shoes.

The nurse helps the patient and family manipulate the home environment to improve the patient's access to bathroom facilities whenever such improvements are feasible. The patient's mobility and access to bathroom facilities are particularly likely to be impaired at night because of the patient's disorientation upon awakening from sleep and poor lighting in the home or bathroom. The nurse may help the patient obtain a bedside urinal or commode to eliminate the need to get up and maneuver to the bathroom. For men a hand-held urinal may be sufficient. For women a bedside commode is a viable option; it should have four sturdy legs with rubber pads that prevent the commode from sliding when it is placed on the floor. The commode should be equipped with arm rails that the patient can use to help seat herself on the toilet and legs that can be adjusted to a proper height for transfers from the bed to the commode and back. The nurse encourages the patient and family to provide adequate lighting in corridors and bathroom facilities. The nurse also helps the patient identify strategies for overcoming such environmental barriers to the bathroom as stairs or throw rugs.

The individual who must use an assistive device such as a wheelchair or walker may need assistance in physically altering his or her home to provide for increased mobility. Assistance may include widening the door to provide access for the wheelchair or walker or installing an extension to raise the toilet seat for easier transfers. Hand-rails may be necessary to facilitate transfers. A rehabilitation specialist may be consulted for assistance when environmental modifications are necessary.

Deficits in Dexterity. Deficits in dexterity may also influence continence. The patient with a neuropathic bladder may experience weakness of one or both hands because of cerebrovascular accident or spinal cord injury. Nursing management focuses on assisting the patient with strategies for overcoming these deficits. The nurse selects equipment with the patient's strengths and limitations in mind and may consult physical or occupational therapists for the assistive devices needed for the patient's bladder management program.

People who manage their bladders by spontaneous voiding may also be affected by limited dexterity. Clothing may be modified so that fewer fine-motor movements are necessary when these patients prepare to void. For example, zippers are easier to manipulate than buttons, and Velcro fasteners are even

---

INTERVENTIONS FOR PATIENTS WITH INCONTINENCE

I. Stress incontinence
   A. Pelvic floor exercises
   B. Pharmacotherapy
      1. Alpha-sympathomimetic agents
      2. Imipramine
      3. Estrogen agents
   C. Pessary devices
   D. Surgical restoration of urethrovesical anatomy
   E. Surgical procedures to increase urethral resistance
II. Instability incontinence
   A. Urge incontinence
      1. Elimination of bladder irritants
      2. Prompted voiding schedule
      3. Bladder drill therapy
      4. Fluid control regimen
      5. Pharmacotherapy
         1. Antispasmodic agents
         2. Anticholinergic agents
      6. Pharmacologic paralysis with clean intermittent catheterization
      7. Electrostimulation of the pelvic floor
      8. Biofeedback therapy
      9. Augmentation cystoplasty
   B. Reflex incontinence
      1. Pharmacologic paralysis with clean intermittent catheterization
      2. Reflex voiding program with containment device
      3. Augmentation cystoplasty
III. Overflow incontinence (urinary retention)
   A. Prompted voiding
      1. Double voiding
      2. Fluid control program
   B. Clean intermittent catheterization
   C. Indwelling catheter
   D. Pharmacotherapy (alpha-adrenergic blocking agents)
IV. Continual incontinence
   A. Correction of cause
   B. Containment and skin protection
V. Functional incontinence
   A. Measures to improve mobility
   B. Measures to maximize dexterity
   C. Measures to enhance mentation and motivation

easier to manipulate than zippers. Patients with limited hand dexterity that affects continence are also advised not to wear too many layers of clothing or underwear.

Altered Mentation and Motivation. Altered mentation may profoundly affect urinary continence. Patients may lack the motivation or orientation to control bladder elimination. In managing the patient with altered mentation, it is critical that the nurse first identify other factors that are contributing to the incontinence, such as organic disease, issues of mobility and access, and the like. After the patient has been assessed carefully, management may consist of a schedule of prompted voiding. The nursing staff or caregiver is asked to help the patient to the bathroom or bedside commode and to encourage the patient to void every 2 hours. The caregiver maintains a voiding diary that documents the amount of urine voided, any evidence of incontinence, and observations regarding the patient's orientation, behavior, and response to the toileting program. When this simple strategy fails to resolve the incontinence, consultation with the urologist and mental health specialist is indicated. Interventions for patients with various types of incontinence are outlined in the box on p. 111.

SURGERY FOR MANAGEMENT OF URINARY INCONTINENCE

The role of surgery in the management of urinary incontinence has evolved during the past 50 years.[3] Surgery may be considered when less invasive forms of management, including behavior modification and pharmacologic therapy, have failed. Surgery is indicated only after a complete urologic evaluation of the patient has been performed, including radiographic and urodynamic studies as necessary. An understanding of the pathophysiology of urine loss and the selection of an appropriate operative procedure are the keys to successful surgical correction of incontinence.[57]

Stress Incontinence Related to Pelvic Floor Relaxation

Stress urinary incontinence is the leakage of small amounts of urine with transient increases in intra-abdominal pressure, as may occur with a cough or a sneeze. Stress incontinence is most common in women and is usually caused by weakness of the pelvic floor muscles, which leads to anatomic displacement of the bladder neck and urethra into the vagina during stress maneuvers. Surgical treatment of this condition is designed to relocate the bladder neck to a relatively fixed intra-abdominal position. Many surgical procedures can accomplish this goal. Surgical procedures for patients with incontinence are outlined in the box on p. 113. The most commonly performed procedures are suprapubic repairs or combined suprapubic and transvaginal repairs.

SURGICAL PROCEDURES FOR PATIENTS WITH URINARY INCONTINENCE

I. Procedures for stress urinary incontinence of anatomic origin
  A. Suprapubic procedures
    1. Marshall-Marchetti-Krantz procedure
    2. Burch colposuspension
    3. Anterior urethropexy
  B. Combined suprapubic and transvaginal procedures
    1. Modified Pereyra bladder neck suspension
    2. Stamey procedure
    3. Gittes procedure

II. Procedures for stress urinary incontinence secondary to intrinsic sphincter dysfunction
  A. Pubovaginal sling procedure
  B. Periurethral injection of Teflon or collagen
  C. Artificial urinary sphincter implant

III. Procedures for incontinence related to bladder dysfunction
  A. Urinary diversion
  B. Bladder augmentation
  C. Cystolysis
  D. Sacral rhizotomy
  E. Pelvic nerve stimulation

Anterior Urethropexy. The anterior urethropexy is a suprapubic procedure designed to correct the most common form of stress urinary incontinence in women.[53] The patient is given a general or a spinal anesthetic and is placed in a supine or "frog-legged" position (Fig. 4-1). A Foley catheter is placed transurethrally. A low abdominal transverse incision is made to gain access to the retropubic space. The bladder neck and urethra are identified. Absorbable supporting sutures are then placed in the anterior wall of the urethra and suspended to the periosteum of the pubic bone (Fig. 4-2). The Foley catheter is usually removed on the fifth postoperative day. If the patient is unable to void when the catheter is removed, she is either treated with a temporary indwelling catheter or taught to perform clean intermittent catheterization until spontaneous voiding occurs.

Modified Pereyra Bladder Neck Suspension. The modified Pereyra bladder neck suspension as described by Raz is an example of a combined suprapubic and transvaginal repair.[35] The patient is given a general or a spinal anesthetic and is placed in a modified lithotomy position. An inverted U-shaped incision is made in the anterior vaginal wall, and through this incision permanent supporting sutures that incorporate the vaginal wall and endopelvic fascia are placed laterally. Using a ligature carrier the surgeon transfers the sutures to a suprapubic position through a small abdominal incision made above the sym-

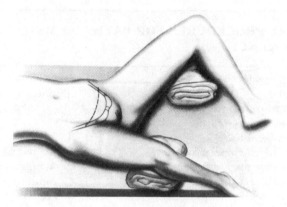

Fig. 4-1 Position of patient and incision for anterior urethropexy. (From Siegel S and Montague D: Surgery for stress incontinence. In Novick A, Streem S, and Pontes J, eds: Stewart's operative urology, ed 2, vol 2, Baltimore, 1989, Williams & Wilkins.)

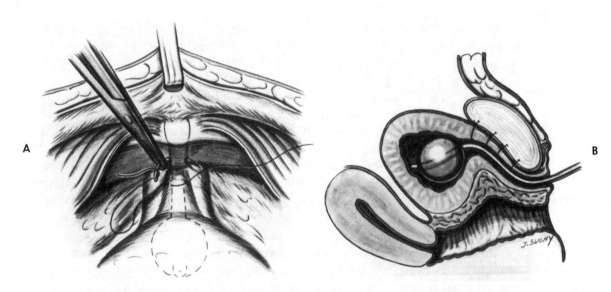

Fig. 4-2 **A,** Anterior urethropexy. Suspending sutures are placed through the anterior wall of the urethra and secured to the periosteum of the symphysis pubis. **B,** Anterior urethropexy. Sagittal view demonstrates elevation of bladder neck and urethra achieved during anterior urethropexy. (From Siegel S and Montague D: Surgery for stress incontinence. In Novick A, Streem S, and Pontes J, eds: Stewart's operative urology, ed 2, vol 2, Baltimore, 1989, Williams & Wilkins.)

physis pubis (Fig. 4-3). Next, the sutures are anchored to the abdominal rectus fascia, thus elevating the bladder neck to an intra-abdominal position. A Foley catheter and vaginal pack are placed at the conclusion of surgery and are removed on the first postoperative day. The patient is taught to perform intermittent catheterization and may discontinue catheterization as soon as her residual urine volumes are less than 100 ml. Approximately one half of patients are able to void within 3 to 5 days; the remainder require intermittent catheterization for a short time.

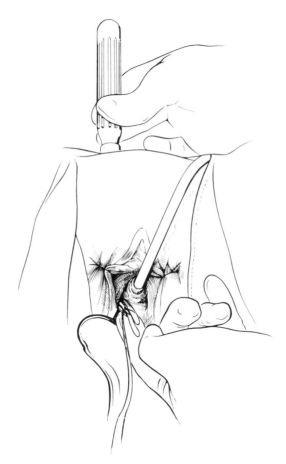

Fig. 4-3   Modified Pereyra bladder neck suspension. Suspending sutures are placed on either side of bladder neck through vaginal incision. Ends of sutures are then transferred to suprapubic area with ligature carrier. (From Siegel S and Montague D: Surgery for stress incontinence. In Novick A, Streem S, and Pontes J, eds: Stewart's operative urology, ed 2, vol 2, Baltimore, 1989, Williams & Wilkins.)

In general, suprapubic repair and combined suprapubic and transvaginal repair are equally effective procedures: approximately 90% of patients with stress incontinence are cured.[55] The primary advantage of the combined procedure is that the potential morbidity associated with the more extensive retropubic dissection performed during the suprapubic procedure can be avoided. Another advantage of the combined repair is that the surgeon can correct coexisting forms of pelvic prolapse such as procidentia, cystocele, rectocele, and prolapse of the vaginal vault.

Stress Incontinence Related to Intrinsic Sphincter Dysfunction

The anatomic displacement of a normal bladder neck and urethra is the cause of stress incontinence in most women. In a few men and women a dysfunctional intrinsic sphincter mechanism is the cause of urine loss. In these patients, repositioning the incompetent bladder neck and urethra will not correct the incontinence; a procedure designed to provide compression of the urethra, thereby increasing urethral resistance, must be employed. Procedures that accomplish this goal include the pubovaginal sling procedure,[39] periurethral injection of Teflon or collagen,[42,52] and the implantation of an artificial urinary sphincter.[18,50]

Pubovaginal Sling Procedure. For the pubovaginal sling procedure, the patient is given a general or a spinal anesthetic and is placed in the modified lithotomy position. A transverse abdominal incision is made, and a strip of anterior rectus fascia is harvested. The fascial defect is then closed, and the fascial sling is positioned around the bladder neck through a midline vaginal incision (Fig. 4-4). The limbs of the sling are then pulled through the retropubic space and anchored to the anterior rectus fascia above the pubic bone.[39] The tension on the sling should be sufficient to obstruct the urethral outlet during rest, yet allow for voluntary voiding. When the patient performs a stress maneuver, the abdominal muscles are tightened, thus tightening the sling and preventing stress incontinence. A suprapubic tube and Foley catheter are left in place along with a vaginal pack. The vaginal pack and urethral Foley catheter are removed on the first postoperative day, and the patient is allowed to void. If the patient is unable to void immediately, the residual urine is evacuated through the suprapubic tube. Most patients are able to urinate to completion within several weeks after this operation.

Periurethral Injection. Periurethral injection of collagen[52] or Teflon[42] also accomplishes the goal of increasing urethral resistance. In this procedure the patient is given a general or a spinal anesthetic. The surgeon uses a cystoscope to visualize the urethral lumen and places a needle beneath the urethral wall. The material is injected circumferentially until the lumen appears to be ob-

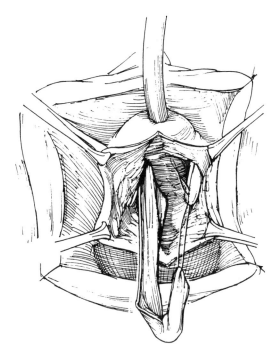

Fig. 4-4 Pubovaginal sling. Fascial sling is placed underneath bladder neck, and limbs of sling are transferred suprapubically, where they are anchored to rectus fascia. (From Hinman F Jr: Atlas of urologic surgery, Philadelphia, 1989, WB Saunders Co.)

structed. Periurethral injection can be used for men with postprostatectomy incontinence secondary to external sphincter injury.[28] The damaged sphincter may appear through the cystoscope as a keyhole deformity. This damaged area can be built up with the injected material to increase resistance and restore continence. Local anesthesia can be used for periurethral injections in outpatients. Frequently the procedure must be repeated after several months to achieve continence. Currently the main limitations of periurethral injection involve the material used: the potential long-term health risks associated with Teflon are unknown, and it appears that collagen may be reabsorbed over time. Neither of these materials is currently approved by the Food and Drug Administration for use in the the urinary tract.

Artificial Urinary Sphincter Implant. A third alternative for management of intrinsic sphincteric incompetence is the implantation of an artificial urinary sphincter.[18,50]

Indications. Candidates for the artificial sphincter include those with neurogenic sphincter incompetence (for example, patients with spina bifida, spinal cord injury, or multiple sclerosis) and those with structural sphincter incompetence (for example, patients who are incontinent after prostatectomy or patients with epispadias or exstrophy). Candidates or caregivers must have the mobility to toilet, the dexterity to manipulate the device, and the motivation for surgery and lifelong follow-up. Vesicoureteral reflux and hyperreflexia, if present, must be amenable to surgical correction or medical management. Implantation of the sphincter is contraindicated in the presence of progressive urologic disease, urinary tract infection, or bacteriuria.[15]

Description of device and implantation. The artificial urinary sphincter (AMS model 800) has three components: a cuff, a pressure-regulating balloon, and a control pump. The components are connected by silicone tubing (Fig. 4-5). The cuff is placed at the bladder neck (or bulbous urethra in older men) and is designed to occlude the urethra when inflated (Fig. 4-6). Several cuff sizes are available; appropriate fit of the cuff, determined by measuring the placement site during surgery, is critical to the effectiveness of the device.[15,20]

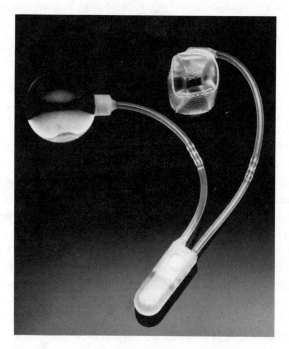

Fig. 4-5 AUS (AMS 800). (Courtesy American Medical Systems, Inc., Minnetonka, Minn.)

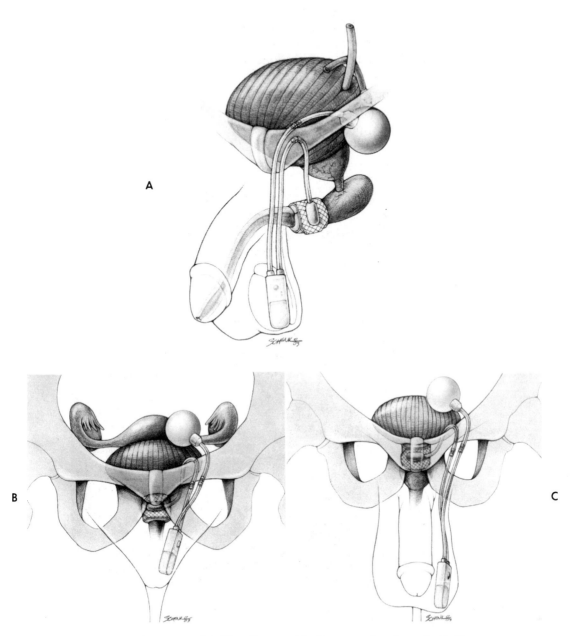

Fig. 4-6 **A,** Placement of AUS cuff around bulbous urethra in male. **B,** Placement of AUS in female. Cuff is placed around bladder neck, balloon is placed in prevesical space, and pump is placed in labia. **C,** Placement of AUS in male. Cuff is placed around bladder neck, balloon is placed in prevesical space, and pump is placed in scrotum. (Courtesy American Medical Systems, Inc., Minnetonka, Minn.)

The pressure-regulating balloon is placed intra-abdominally in the prevesical space; the balloon regulates the closing pressure of the cuff around the urethra (Fig. 4-6). Balloons are available in a range of sizes that deliver various pressures; the balloon size that provides enough pressure to occlude the urethral cuff without impairing urethral blood supply should be selected. The size of the balloon is determined by cuff size and characteristics of the tissue underlying the cuff. The cuff and balloon are usually filled with an iodine-based radiopaque solution (unless the patient has an allergy to iodine), which permits radiologic visualization of the device.[15]

The control pump is surgically placed in the labia for females or the scrotum for males (Fig. 4-6). Compression of the pump diverts fluid from the cuff to the balloon and results in cuff deflation; the patient is then able to void or catheterize through the open urethra. The cuff then self-inflates over a period of 3 to 5 minutes, thus reestablishing continence (Fig. 4-7, *1* and *2*).[15]

The device is usually left deactivated (cuff deflated) immediately after surgery to allow for healing of the periurethral tissue. It may also be deactivated whenever indwelling catheterization is necessary. The device is deactivated by depressing a small poppet button on the side of the control pump after the cuff

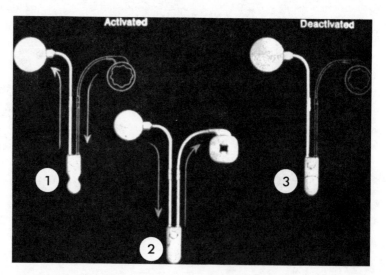

Fig. 4-7   *1,* AUS mimics normal urination and control. To void, pump is squeezed several times until it feels flat. Squeezing moves fluid out of cuff, through tubing, and into balloon. *2,* Fluid automatically returns to cuff, again closing urethra and restoring continence. *3,* AUS can be deactivated by pumping fluid out of cuff and then pressing button on control pump to "lock" fluid in balloon. (From Faller N and Vinson R: J Enterost Ther 12[1]:12, 1985.)

has been deflated. This maneuver locks fluid in the balloon (Fig. 4-7, 3). The device is reactivated by firmly squeezing the control pump.[51]

Effectiveness. Implantation of the artificial urinary sphincter improves continence for most patients. In a recent series of 304 adults, 73% were "socially continent" (dry or requiring less than three pads per day to contain leakage) after implantation; only 7% reported persistent wetness.[51] However, a significant number of patients (20% in the series of 304 adults) require device removal or revision; removal is most often necessitated by erosion, infection, or a combination of the two. Scott also reported decreasing success over time, that is, only 55% of the patients who were initially "totally dry" maintained that level of continence.[51] Scott attributed this decreasing success to atrophy of the tissue under the cuff, which alters the fit of the cuff.

Preoperative and postoperative management. Preoperative workup is directed toward identification of any contraindications to artificial urinary sphincter implantation and includes a history and physical, an intravenous pyelogram, cystoscopy, a voiding cystourethrogram, a cystometrogram and electromyogram, studies of urinary flow and postvoid residual volume, and psychologic evaluation. Once testing confirms the patient's candidacy for an artificial sphinctor, the patient is shown a sample of an artificial sphincter. Patients with low voiding pressures, high postvoid residual volumes, or inadequate urinary flow rates are instructed in clean intermittent catheterization at this time.[15]

When the patient is admitted for surgery, a urine specimen is obtained and examined for any urinary tract infection or bacteriuria. Any infection must be treated aggressively.[51] The patient is questioned regarding any allergy to iodine.

Postoperatively, urine output is monitored and the wound is observed for drainage and signs of infection. Before discharge the individual is given both verbal and written instructions for home care that include the topics of wound care, signs and symptoms of wound infection and appropriate response, catheter care (if the patient is sent home with an indwelling catheter), and device management (for example, the correct positioning of the control pump into the scrotum or labia 1 to 3 times daily).[15]

Six weeks postoperatively the individual is taught how to deflate the cuff. (Depending on urine volume and flow rate, the patient may need to deflate the cuff twice for each void.) Frequency of urination or catheterization is determined by sensations of fullness or by a schedule based on intake. The patient is given a medical identification card and an application for an identifying (Medic-Alert) bracelet or necklace, and the importance of medical identification is stressed. Patients must be taught to recognize and respond to signs of complications such as infection and erosion. Patients are also instructed in any necessary modifications of normal activity (for example, modified seating for bicycle riding or modifications for other sports).[15]

Urinary Incontinence Caused by Bladder Dysfunction

A dysfunctional bladder can also cause urinary incontinence. Volitional control of urination requires low-pressure storage of urine. Urinary incontinence secondary to bladder instability or hyperreflexia occurs when uninhibited detrusor contractions cause bladder pressure to rise above urethral pressure and result in urine loss. Frequently, bladder instability is managed with anticholinergic medications that diminish the force of uninhibited contractions. When such treatment fails or the medications cannot be tolerated, surgical management is an alternative. Appropriate surgical techniques for the management of this condition include diversion of the urine away from the bladder via an ileal conduit or a continent urinary reservoir, or augmentation of the bladder with an intestinal segment.

Urinary Diversion. Construction of an ileal conduit is a major abdominal surgery. The patient must be hospitalized preoperatively to receive a mechan-

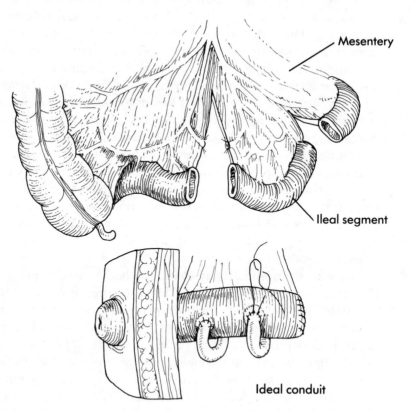

Mesentery

Ileal segment

Ideal conduit

Fig. 4-8   Construction of ileal conduit. Ureters are anastomosed to proximal end of conduit, and stoma is fashioned from distal end. (From Broadwell D: Principles of ostomy care, St Louis, 1982, Mosby–Year Book.)

ical bowel prep and intravenous antibiotics. A segment of the terminal ileum is isolated through a midline abdominal incision. The ureters, which are removed from the bladder, are anastomosed to the proximal end of the ileal segment, and the distal end is brought to the abdominal wall to form a stoma (Fig. 4-8).

The management of patients with urostomies has been greatly facilitated by the evolution of the ET nursing specialty. Disadvantages of an ileal conduit include the deterioration of the upper tracts, which is known to occur over time, and the need to wear an external urine collection device, which many patients find undesirable.

Urinary diversion can also be achieved with a continent urinary reservoir such as the Indiana reservoir,[48] the Koch urostomy,[33] or the Mitrofanoff pouch.[11] Patients managed with a continent urinary reservoir generally do not require an appliance and are able to empty the reservoir by catheterization at discreet intervals. Additionally, antirefluxing anastomoses of the ureters are included to protect the upper urinary tracts.

Bladder Augmentation. Surgical augmentation of a small-capacity, hyperreflexic bladder is an alternative to urinary diversion.[36] Patients having bladder augmentation must be hospitalized preoperatively for bowel preparation and

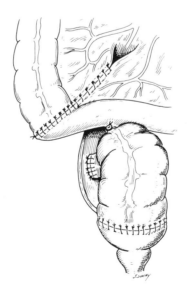

Fig. 4-9 Bladder augmentation. Ileocecal segment of colon has been used to increase bladder storage capacity. (From Novick A: Augmentation cystoplasty. In Novick A, Streem S, and Pontes J, eds: Stewart's operative urology, ed 2, vol 2, Baltimore, 1989, Williams & Wilkins.)

antibiotic prophylaxis. After the patient has been given a general anesthetic, a midline incision is made and a segment of intestine, such as the ascending colon, is isolated on its vascular pedicle. The intestinal segment is fashioned as a patch to augment the bladder (Fig. 4-9). In the case of an associated sphincter dysfunction, the augmentation can be performed in conjunction with a procedure designed to increase urethral resistance. Prolonged use of suprapubic tubes and Foley catheters is usually necessary to prevent bladder distention until healing is complete. Because the intestinal patch produces mucus, intermittent bladder irrigation may be necessary to prevent obstruction from a mucus plug. Other possible complications include bowel obstruction, anastomotic complications, and urinary fistulae. Many patients who have augmentation for a neurogenic bladder require long-term intermittent catheterization to empty the bladder efficiently.

Other surgical procedures designed to treat a dysfunctional bladder involve interruption of the bladder's neurologic input. This interruption can be accomplished by means of a sacral rhizotomy or cystolysis.[19] Newer techniques that involve pelvic nerve stimulation by way of percutaneous wire implants are now being developed.[58] Although the use of cystolysis has fallen into disfavor, sacral rhizotomy used alone or in conjunction with pelvic nerve stimulation may prove to be effective in some patients.

PHARMACOLOGIC OPTIONS FOR MANAGEMENT OF URINARY INCONTINENCE

Many drugs have been implicated as contributing factors in dysfunctional voiding states and urinary incontinence (Table 4-1). Conversely, several drugs have been used effectively in the management of urinary incontinence, although most drugs currently being used have not been studied in well-designed clinical trials. Medications can be employed to increase or decrease bladder contractility and to increase or decrease urethral resistance. Drugs commonly used in the management of urinary incontinence are discussed in this section, with attention to the mechanisms of action, contraindications, and common side effects. Pharmacologic manipulation is most effective when employed as a *component* of a bladder management program; patient education regarding prescribed medications is an important aspect of that program.

Bladder Instability (Urge Incontinence, Reflex Incontinence)

Several available drugs reduce uninhibited (involuntary) bladder contractions, thereby increasing bladder capacity. Since one attendant risk of this type of drug is urinary retention, bladder outlet obstruction or impaired detrusor contractility is a possible contraindication to use of these agents and should be considered in patient evaluation.

Table 4-1 Medications that may affect continence

Type of drug	Potential effects on continence
Diuretics	Polyuria, frequency, urgency
Anticholinergics	Urinary retention, overflow incontinence, impaction
Psychotropics	
Antidepressants	Anticholinergic effects, sedation
Antipsychotics	Anticholinergic effects, sedation, rigidity, immobility
Sedatives and hypnotics	Sedation, delirium, immobility, muscle relaxation
Narcotic analgesics	Urinary retention, fecal impaction, sedation, delirium
Alpha-adrenergic blockers	Urethral relaxation
Alpha-adrenergic agonists	Urinary retention
Beta-adrenergic agonists	Urinary retention
Calcium channel blockers	Urinary retention
Alcohol	Polyuria, frequency, urgency, sedation, immobility, delirium

Anticholinergic Drugs. Cholinergic receptors are thought to mediate not only normal bladder contractions but also the major component of contractions in hyperactive bladders. Atropine and other anticholinergic drugs are known to produce an almost complete paralysis of the normal bladder when injected intravenously.[2] Anticholinergic agents inhibit detrusor contractility and may delay and reduce the amplitude of involuntary contractions, thus increasing functional bladder capacity.

Propantheline (Pro-Banthine). Propantheline is most commonly used in the treatment of urge incontinence or stress incontinence with detrusor instability. The usual dosage is 15 to 30 mg by mouth three times a day. Propantheline should be used with caution in patients with glaucoma, heart disease, hiatal hernia, high blood pressure, intestinal blockage, kidney disease, liver disease, lung disease, myasthenia gravis, enlarged prostate gland, thyroid disease, ulcerative colitis, or urinary retention. Common side effects include dry mouth, dry eyes, blurred vision, increased intraocular pressure, and constipation. In higher doses, especially in elderly patients receiving other drugs with anticholinergic effects (for example, antidepressants or antipsychotics), propantheline can cause delirium, mental confusion, orthostatic hypotension, and increased heart rate. Because of these side effects, elderly patients may be managed with half the therapeutic dose.[47] Side effects of propantheline usually decrease as the patient becomes accustomed to the medication.

PATIENT INSTRUCTIONS

Because propantheline can decrease sweating and heat release from the body, the patient should be cautioned against becoming overheated: hot baths, showers, saunas, and strenuous exercise in hot weather should be avoided. In addition, the patient should be cautioned to avoid activities that require mental alertness (for example, driving or operating machinery) if the medication causes dizziness, drowsiness, or blurred vision. To prevent constipation, the patient can increase the amount of fiber in his or her diet, exercise, and increase fluid intake. Mouth dryness can be relieved by chewing sugarless gum or sucking on hard candy or ice chips. Artificial tear solutions may be used for relief of dry eyes.[41,54]

Direct Smooth-Muscle Relaxants. Smooth-muscle relaxants act directly on the bladder muscle to reduce its contractility and to produce an antispasmodic effect; they have a mild anticholinergic effect as well.

Oxybutynin (Ditropan). A pronounced direct muscle relaxant effect has been attributed to oxybutynin, whereas its level of anticholinergic action is considered to be moderate to high. Oxybutynin exhibits one fifth of the anticholinergic effect of atropine but 4 to 10 times the antispasmodic activity.[47] Oxybutynin has a well-documented therapeutic effect in detrusor hyperreflexia, although it is also associated with a high incidence of side effects. Oxybutynin is indicated in the management of patients with instability (urge or reflex) incontinence. The recommended dosage is 2.5 to 5.0 mg by mouth two or three times a day. Side effects, cautions, and patient instructions are the same as those for propantheline.[41,54]

Dicyclomine (Bentyl). Dicyclomine acts to diminish involuntary bladder contractions by both anticholinergic actions and direct smooth-muscle relaxant effects. Dosage is 10 to 20 mg by mouth three times a day. Side effects are generally anticholinergic: blurred vision, dry mouth, nose, and throat, headache, increased sensitivity to light, insomnia, and confusion are most commonly seen. Contraindications and patient instructions are the same as those for propantheline.[41,54]

Flavoxate (Urispas). Flavoxate counteracts smooth-muscle spasm by cholinergic blockade and by a direct relaxant effect on the muscle; in addition, it provides some local anesthesia and analgesia. The clinical effectiveness of flavoxate in the control of detrusor instability (reduction of urinary frequency and urge incontinence) has been studied in both open and controlled investigations, and varying rates of success have been reported.[2] The recommended dosage for adults is 100 to 200 mg by mouth three or four times daily; the dosage should be reduced as the patient's condition improves. The drug is contraindicated in patients with pyloric or duodenal obstruction, obstructive intestinal lesions or ileus, achalasia, gastrointestinal hemorrhage, or obstructive uropathies of the lower urinary tract. Flavoxate should be used with caution in patients with glaucoma. Side effects include nausea and vomiting, dry mouth, nervousness, vertigo, headache, mental confusion (especially in elderly patients), blurred vision, and tachycardia. Patient instructions should include cautions against driving or performing hazardous activities should dizziness or drowsiness occur.[41,54]

Imipramine (Tofranil). Imipramine produces marked systemic anticholinergic actions; however, the mechanism that produces its effect on the bladder has not been established. Imipramine exerts a marked direct inhibitory effect on the detrusor; its anticholinergic effect on bladder muscle seems weak. Imipramine is the only antidepressant that has been widely used for the treatment of bladder instability and for the treatment of nocturnal enuresis in children. The usual dose is 25 to 50 mg by mouth three times daily. Contraindications include convulsive disorders, prostate hypertrophy, and the recovery phase of myocardial infarction. Cautions, side effects, and patient instructions are the same as those for anticholinergic agents (for example, propantheline); in addition, the patient must be observed for and counseled about possible postural hypotension, sedation, and ventricular arrhythmias. In elderly patients the use of imipramine must be monitored closely because of its systemic anticholinergic effects.[41,54]

Calcium Channel Blockers. These agents are used in the clinical management of cardiovascular and hypertensive disease. They have a depressant effect on the bladder as well; however, they have not been studied rigorously for the treatment of instability incontinence. When these drugs are being considered for the treatment of cardiac disease, their effects on the bladder must be kept in mind, that is, both the potential benefit and the risk of urinary retention must be considered.

Calcium channel antagonists inhibit the cellular influx of calcium in smooth muscle. Inhibition of calcium influx may reduce involuntary detrusor contractions. In tests using human bladder muscle, nifedipine (Procardia) was shown in vitro to relax the muscle samples that had contracted in response to contractile agents and to decrease the contractile response in pretreated tissue.[47] These authors also demonstrated that in patients with urge incontinence the administration of nifedipine increased the volume of residual urine; this increase in residual volume suggests a decrease in bladder contractility.[47] The role of calcium channel blockers in the management of urinary incontinence has not yet been clearly defined.

Stress Incontinence

Alpha-Adrenergic Agonists. These sympathomimetic drugs are used in the treatment of stress incontinence related to sphincter weakness; they have been most effective in cases of mild to moderate stress incontinence. The smooth muscle of the urethra contains both cholinergic (muscarinic) and adrenergic (sympathetic) receptors. Stimulation of the adrenergic receptors causes contraction of the smooth muscle and produces an increase in urethral pressure. Frequently alpha-adrenergic agonists are used in combination with other drugs or treatments (for example, pelvic floor exercises) to control stress incontinence.

Pseudoephedrine (Sudafed). The oral dosage of pseudoephedrine for the treatment of stress incontinence is 15 to 30 mg three times daily. Sympathomimetics should be used with caution in patients with hypertension, hyperthyroidism, diabetes mellitus, cardiovascular disease, coronary artery disease, ischemic heart disease, increased intraocular pressure, or prostatic hypertrophy. Adverse effects associated with these drugs include mental confusion, convulsions, and hallucinations, especially in elderly patients. Less serious side effects include anxiety, tremors, restlessness, headache, lightheadedness, dizziness, drowsiness, insomnia, arrhythmias, and palpitations.[41] Patients should be cautioned against driving or operating machinery if dizziness or drowsiness occurs and instructed to notify the physician of heart irregularities or palpitations.[54]

Phenylpropanolamine (Ornade). The oral dose of phenylpropanolamine is 75 mg twice daily. Adverse effects, cautions, and patient instructions are the same as those for pseudoephedrine.

Conjugated Estrogens (Premarin). Several studies have reported beneficial effects of estrogens in patients with stress urinary incontinence, including proliferation of the urethral mucosa with consequent improvement in the mucosal "seal" and increased urethral resistance.[2] Treatment with estrogens has also been reported to increase the effect of alpha-adrenergic stimulation on the urethral smooth muscle.[47]

Both oral and topical estrogens have been used for the treatment of stress incontinence and urge incontinence associated with atrophic vaginitis. The oral dose is 0.625 mg of conjugated estrogen per day; the topical dose is 0.5 to 1.0 g per application. Estrogen administration has been associated with an increased incidence of endometrial cancer, hypertension, and gallstones; these risks as well as the benefits of treatment, should be considered in the long-term administration of estrogen. Other side effects associated with estrogen administration include bloating, fluid retention, change in sexual desire, depression, diarrhea, dizziness, headache, loss of appetite, nausea, and vomiting. Patient instructions include the correct administration (route and schedule) of estrogen and the management and reporting of side effects.[41,54]

Overflow Incontinence (Retention)

Overflow (paradoxical) incontinence occurs when the bladder does not empty effectively. The primary cause of retention may be related to insufficient detrusor contractility; retention can also be caused by urethral obstruction that creates increased resistance to outflow.

Cholinergic Agents. Detrusor contractility is mediated by stimulation of cholinergic (parasympathetic) receptors; drugs that stimulate these receptors can improve bladder contraction and facilitate bladder emptying for patients with impaired detrusor contractility.

Bethanechol (Urecholine). Several clinical studies suggest that cholinergic agents such as bethanechol are not effective in reducing the volume of residual urine. However, bethanechol is thought to be useful for some patients.[47] The dosage is 10 to 30 mg by mouth three times daily. Side effects include bradycardia, hypotension, bronchoconstriction, increased secretion of gastric acid, and gastrointestinal discomfort. Patient instructions include the management of side effects (for example, administration with food or milk to reduce gastrointestinal distress and gradual position changes to minimize postural hypotension) and prompt notification of the physician concerning any serious side effects (for example, severe dizziness or difficulty breathing).

Alpha-Adrenergic Blocking Agents. Alpha-adrenergic receptors in the bladder neck and urethra increase urethral resistance; alpha-adrenergic blocking agents are used to reduce urethral resistance and improve bladder emptying.

Phenoxybenzamine (Dibenzyline). The initial dosage of phenoxybenzamine is 10 mg by mouth daily; the dose may be increased by 10 mg every 4 to 5 days to a recommended maximum dosage of 60 mg daily. Unfortunately, adverse reactions are frequent and severe; they include nasal congestion, miosis, postural hypotension with dizziness, and tachycardia. Less common side effects include drowsiness, fatigue, weakness, lassitude, malaise, confusion, and inhibition of ejaculation. Patient instructions include the avoidance of alcohol, gradual position changes to minimize postural hypotension, and the avoidance of over-the-counter medications not approved by the physician.[41,54]

Prazosin (Minipress). Prazosin has been found to decrease both urethral resistance and residual volumes of urine. The usual dosage is 1 to 2 mg by mouth 3 times daily. Adverse effects include those described for phenoxybenzamine but in a lower incidence. Common side effects include nausea, vomiting, depression, hallucinations, postural hypotension, palpitations, rapid or irregular pulse, and rash.[41] The patient is instructed to take the first dose at bedtime to reduce the dizziness that may occur early in therapy; to avoid over-the-counter preparations (unless approved by the physician), since these agents can interfere with the intended effects of prazosin; and to watch for edema, which can result from the retention of sodium and water.

The nurse's role in the management of any patient taking medications for the treatment of urinary incontinence includes patient education regarding the drug, its correct dose and schedule, and its potential side effects. In addition, the nurse helps monitor the patient's response to the drug in terms of improved bladder control.

MANAGEMENT OF INTRACTABLE INCONTINENCE

After thorough assessment and diagnostic evaluation, an appropriate bladder management program is devised for each patient. Containment devices and skin protection may be necessary for the patient with total (continual) incontinence unless and until the underlying problem can be corrected; containment may also be appropriate for some patients with instability (reflex or urge) incontinence, and, at times, for the patient with stress incontinence. Containment devices can be used to manage the incontinence during the workup, if initial treatments are ineffective or if the patient is unable or unwilling to participate in treatment.

Containment devices can be categorized as compression devices, collection systems, indwelling catheters, and containment products. To maintain intact and healthy tissue, scrupulous skin care is imperative no matter which containment device is chosen.

Compression Devices

Clamp or Cuff for Men. Compression devices for men include the penile clamp and the compression cuff (Fig. 4-10). The penile clamp is a metallic or plastic

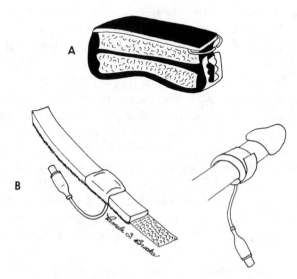

Fig. 4-10   A, Penile clamp. **B,** Compression cuff.

hinged device with an inner lining of foam. The clamp is closed around the penis with enough pressure to occlude the urethra and prevent urine leakage. An inflatable compression cuff is also available. This cuff encircles the penis, and when the inflatable portion is filled with air, it compresses the urethra and prevents urine flow. These devices are released every 2 to 4 hours to allow for bladder emptying and maintenance of tissue integrity; they should not be worn at night. The penile clamp and the compression cuff are useful when a damaged urinary sphincter causes continuous dribbling of urine.[5] These devices should be used only by mentally competent, motivated, and manually dextrous individuals.[5,7] Complications include urinary tract infection, pressure necrosis, and tissue damage.[5]

Pessaries for Women. Incidental urethral compression can improve urinary control in certain women with stress incontinence and can be accomplished by the use of pessaries.[5,44] Pessaries may be indicated for patients who do not respond to pelvic floor exercises and who are not candidates for surgical correction.[57] Pessaries are soft rubber devices of various sizes and shapes; a pessary is inserted into the vagina to support tissue structures and produce a more normal vesicourethral anatomy (Fig. 4-11). A gynecologic examination before use is mandatory. Patients must be taught how to insert and remove the device and how to clean it; they must also be taught the importance of tissue rest. If

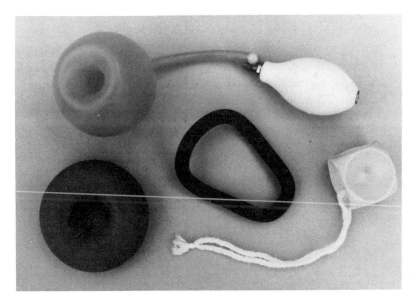

Fig. 4-11 Examples of pessaries. (From Droegemueller W: Comprehensive gynecology, St Louis, 1987, Mosby–Year Book, Inc.)

the patient cannot remove and reinsert the pessary herself, a follow-up program must be devised for routine removal, cleansing, and reinsertion of the device by a professional health care provider. The patient should be examined every 2 to 3 months: the individual's proficiency in the use of the device should be evaluated, and the examiner should also assess signs and symptoms of urinary tract infection, voiding difficulties, vaginal discharge, or discomfort.[5,38,59]

External Collection Systems

Systems for Men. A variety of external collection systems is available for men and includes urinals, condom catheters, and pouching systems. A support urinal consists of a latex sheath that fits over the penis and is held in place with either a cloth support or rubber straps. The pubic pressure urinal has a semirigid flange; the flange provides firmness and pressure to the pubic area, which causes the penis to push forward into the latex sheath. The pubic pressure urinal is particularly useful for the patient with a retracted penis.[4]

A condom catheter consists of a thin latex sheath that is secured to the penis by means of adhesive strips, external straps, or a self-adhesive inner lining. The secured sheath is connected to a drainage tube that leads to a leg bag or a bedside drainage container. Condom catheters with molding at the connective end are preferable: they prevent kinking and twisting, they are more durable for large-volume voiding, and they hold the tip of the condom away from the penile head, thereby improving drainage.[5] Improved drainage in turn prevents the penis from being continually bathed in urine.

Condom catheters are most effective when the penile skin is clean and dry and the pubic hair is clipped or shaved. Skin sealants (copolymer films) may be used to protect the skin and enhance the adhesion of the sheath to the skin. An appropriately sized condom is placed with care to prevent constriction. These devices are changed daily or every other day so that tissue integrity can be assessed and skin care can be provided. Local complications occasionally develop when condom catheters are used. These complications include erythema, maceration, and ulceration, urethral diverticulum and fistula, pressure ulcers, and penile gangrene.[26,60] These problems can be minimized by careful application of the device. If complications develop, the condom catheter must be removed until healing is complete.

If an individual cannot be fitted with an external (condom) catheter, pouching the penis with a solid wafer skin barrier and urinary pouch may be of benefit. A pouch (Retracted Penis Pouch) designed for the retracted penis is also available (Hollister, Inc., Libertyville, Ill.).

Systems for Women. Historically the success of external collection systems for women has been limited. For nonambulatory women an external pouch with an attached solid wafer skin barrier is available. The aperture of the skin barrier is sized to encompass the vulva, and the pouch is connected to a bedside drainage system.[25]

Other external collection systems for women have provided satisfactory results in some cases. These systems include silicone devices such as the Female Urinary Incontinence System (Hollister, Inc., Libertyville, Ill.) and the Misstique External Urinary Collection (EUC) System for Women (ITW, Deltar/ Diamed, Elk Grove Village, Ill.). These devices are held in position over the urinary meatus by product design or adhesives or both. A support liner or custom undergarment or both must be used with these devices. These devices are worn for gradually increased periods of time, until a maximum wearing time of 24 hours is achieved. Every 24 hours these devices should be removed and cleansed. Before recommending these products, the nurse must ascertain whether the patient has received or will receive any pelvic radiation treatments, because irradiated tissue is more sensitive to adhesives, solvents, and pressure.

Indwelling Catheters

Indications for Use. The indwelling urethral catheter is a treatment of last resort for the long-term management of urinary incontinence; however, in certain instances its use is appropriate. Indications for long-term use of indwelling catheters include the following:

1. The management of pressure ulcers or surgical wounds that cannot heal because of constant contact with urine or, in selected cases, the prevention of skin breakdown
2. Overflow incontinence associated with unresectable obstruction
3. Painful physical movement that prohibits frequent changes of clothing or protective garments
4. Instances in which the patient or the patient's family decides that considerations of dryness and comfort outweigh the risks of urethral catheterization, such as cases of serious or terminal illness.[32,43,60]

Complications. Bacteriuria is universal after catheters have been in place for 30 days or longer.[60,61] Treatment of bacteriuria is usually reserved for patients who become symptomatic, since treatment in asymptomatic patients results in antibiotic-resistant strains of organisms.[60,61] Other, less common complications of indwelling catheter use include purulent epididymitis, scrotal abscess, prostatic abscess, urethral fistula, bladder calculi, vesicoureteral reflux, obstruction, and chronic tubulointerstitial nephritis.[60]

Catheter Type and Size. Once the decision has been made to use urethral catheterization, the type of catheter is determined. Latex catheters are prone to encrustation and are associated with an increased incidence of urethral irritation with long-term use. Catheters coated with silicone or Teflon are less irritating to urethral tissues and less prone to encrustation.[32,61,62] The catheter should be as small as possible; a French size 14 to 16 catheter is used most commonly. A properly inflated balloon with a capacity of 5 to 10 cc is usually adequate. Larger balloons may cause spasms, and underinflation causes leakage around the catheter. To decrease bacterial contamination, a closed system is used.

Indications for Catheter Change. Most authors agree that a routine schedule for catheter change is not beneficial.[12,32,43,61,62] The change interval is individually determined by considering catheter encrustation and patient comfort. Weiss suggested that silicone-coated catheters be changed every 8 to 12 weeks and Teflon-coated catheters be changed monthly.[61] Kniep-Hardy et al. suggested that patients begin with a monthly catheter change; if no grit or encrustation is found when the catheter is removed, the interval between changes can be increased gradually to 6 weeks and then to 8 weeks.[32]

Routine Care. Cleansing of the periurethral area with soap and water each day and after each bowel movement is recommended. Use of antimicrobial cleansers or ointments has not been found to decrease the incidence of bacteriuria.[61]

Encrustation of the catheter can cause blockage with resultant leakage around the catheter. Encrusted material is frequently associated with an alkaline urine. Increasing the acidity of the urine may be helpful; however, acidification of the urine is controversial.[31] Before initiating an acidification program, the nurse should access the patient for any contraindications such as a history of uric acid stones, gout, current treatment with sulfa drugs, and treatment with some chemotherapeutic agents. If acidification of the urine is desirable, acidification measures include adequate daily fluid intake, reduced intake of dairy products and citrus juices, and ascorbic acid intake.

Management of Leakage. Leakage around the catheter may be caused by a catheter or balloon of improper size, encrustations, or bladder spasms. If bladder spasms occur, the nurse should check for fecal impaction or chronic constipation, since pressure on the bladder from a full rectum may trigger the spasm. A regular bowel regimen should alleviate this problem. The patient should also be assessed for concentrated urine and signs and symptoms of a urinary tract infection, since these factors may also cause bladder spasms. The causative factor should then be addressed. The use of anticholinergic drugs or smooth muscle relaxants (for example, oxybutynin or flavoxate) may be necessary.[12,32,61]

Urine Drainage Bags. Urine drainage bags come in a wide variety of sizes, shapes, and styles: leg bags, systems for night drainage, and collectors suspended from the waist. Whatever style is chosen, a free flow of urine must be maintained at all times. As stated previously, the drainage system should be equipped with a nonreturn valve at the inlet and an easily manipulated outlet tap. The drainage system should be rinsed after each use and routinely cleansed with warm, soapy water. (Hot water should be avoided, since it allows the odor of urine to penetrate the drainage system.) After the system is washed, it should be soaked in a vinegar solution or a commercially prepared solution for 10 to 15 minutes and then hung to dry.

In some cases suprapubic catheters are used for long-term bladder drainage.[17,60]

Containment Products

A wide variety of containment products is available. The choice of product depends on many factors,[1,5] which are listed in the box below.

An excellent guide to currently available products is the *Resource Guide of Continence Products and Services,** in which products are listed and briefly described and an index of manufacturers and distributors is provided.

Diapers. Adult diapers are used for patients with leakage of large volumes of urine or for patients with both urinary and fecal incontinence. Diapers may be reusable or disposable. Reusable diapers are made of cloth with a waterproof backing and are pinned together. Disposable diapers should fit snugly and have fitted legs with elastic to prevent leakage. Special features of disposable diapers may include contour fitting, elastic at the waist, external wetness indicators, and reusable tape tags. Some disposable diapers also contain superabsorbent

---

*Available for a fee from HIP (Help for Incontinent People), P.O. Box 544, Union, SC, 29379.

FACTORS TO CONSIDER WHEN CHOOSING A CONTAINMENT PRODUCT	
Quantity of urine per void	Patient preference
Voiding pattern	Product profile beneath clothing
Simplicity of use	Durability (disposable versus reusable products)
Cost of the product	
Availability of the product	Noise level of the product
Patient comfort	Odor control properties

polymers that buffer odors and gel fluid to prevent seepage. Meticulous skin care is a must for individuals who use diapers.

Inserts. Although commercial menstrual products are used by many incontinent women, these products are usually unacceptable because they do not contain urine well. Inserts are absorbent pads contoured to fit inside undergarments and improve urine dispersion. They have a waterproof backing with adhesive strips that affix them to undergarments. Many inserts contain superabsorbent polymers.

Disposable inserts for men are available as drip collectors. These drip collectors are pocket shaped to fit around the penis or cup shaped to include the penis and scrotum (Fig. 4-12). Drip collectors are useful in cases of mild urinary incontinence. Close-fitting underwear, athletic supporters, or mesh briefs hold these inserts in position.

Pads with Straps. A pad with a strap consists of a large, waterproof-backed pad that extends to the waist; the pad is held in position by being buttoned to elastic side straps. These products are used in cases of moderate incontinence, but leakage often occurs when the wearer assumes the recumbent position.

Pads with Pants. Many kinds of pads with pants are available. For adequate containment and comfort, the garment must be properly sized according to either body weight or waist and hip measurements. Most combinations of pad and pant feature a reusable pant with a disposable pad. The pants may be a brief style or may be held in place with elastic, snaps, or Velcro fasteners. When the pad has a waterproof backing, it is used with jersey, cotton, or mesh briefs.

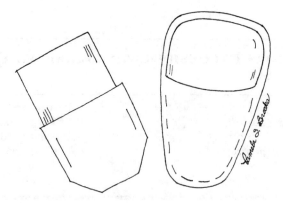

Fig. 4-12   Drip collectors for men.

The pads may contain a superabsorbent polymer; some pads are flushable, which simplifies disposal. Disposable pants have an absorbent crotch with a waterproof exterior. Washable absorbent pants are also available. Plastic pants are unacceptable unless the patient specifically asks to use them.

Underpads. Used to protect the patient's immediate environment (for example, bedding, chairs, and the like), underpads ideally extend beyond the leg and torso and remain soft and dry against the skin. These products are most useful for patients with mild incontinence.[7] Disposable underpads are made of three layers, an upper, nonwoven, liquid-permeable layer, an absorbent layer of cellulose wadding or fluff pulp, and an outer layer that is waterproof. If a pad clings or shreds when it becomes wet or if more than one pad must be used to contain a void, another product may be more suitable.

Reusable underpads have an absorbent cloth layer with a waterproof backing and are available in various sizes. Laundering reusable pads may be a problem in homes without laundry facilities.

Summary. Containment devices can be categorized as compression devices, collection systems, indwelling catheters, and containment products. After patient assessment is complete, appropriate containment devices are selected. Often a period of trial and error is necessary until the most appropriate device for a particular individual is found. The nurse can significantly influence this selection process and help the individual participate to his or her full capability in living and enjoying life.

Skin Care

Routine Care. Once incontinence is apparent, appropriate skin care should be initiated. Keeping the skin dry and intact is of primary importance; a secondary consideration may be a dry bed. Previous or planned radiation treatment to the area is ascertained. Prophylactic skin care is implemented and explained to the patient or family or both. After each incontinent episode the skin is cleansed with water and, if necessary, with a pH-balanced soap, rinsed, and patted dry. A blow dryer on a cool setting may be used to dry the skin. Such devices must be institutionally approved as electrically safe. Commercial cleansers are available and can be used to cleanse the skin frequently without causing dryness or irritation. Some cleansers also have deodorizing properties.

After the skin has been cleansed, a small amount of moisturizing cream is applied as necessary. This cream keeps the skin soft and supple and lubricates the tissue. Creams that contain significant amounts of alcohol should not be used, since alcohol has a drying effect. Topical preparations may be dangerous for irradiated skin; any protocol for skin care should be approved by the radiation oncologist or nurse specialist before it is used on irradiated skin.

Skin Protection. If urine leakage is continuous or skin irritation develops, the skin should be further protected. Skin sealants or moisture barrier ointments may be used. Skin sealants provide a clear, copolymer film to the skin. Many of these are soluble in soap and water and must be reapplied every 12 to 24 hours; the nurse should review specific product information to ensure appropriate use. Moisture barrier ointments should be applied to clean, dry skin and reapplied after each incontinent episode.

Management of Skin Problems. Skin barrier powders or prescription powders may be used to treat skin problems. The powders are dusted onto clean, dry skin; excess powder is brushed away. Sealants may then be used to "seal in" the powder.

Monilial rash *(Candida albicans)* is not uncommon; it is seen as a characteristic patch of erythema containing macules or papules with satellite lesions. Treatment consists of over-the-counter or prescribed antifungal products. These products are available as powders, creams, or ointments. If the tissue is moist and drying is necessary, powders are effective. In cases of incontinence that result in large volumes of urine, creams or ointments may be better vehicles for delivery of medication, since creams and ointments are not washed away as easily as powders. As the monilial rash heals, it may become dry and flaky; if this condition occurs, a cream-based antifungal product can be used to lubricate the tissues. Severe skin problems may necessitate referral to a physician.

Cleansers, moisturizing creams, and moisture barrier ointments are available from a variety of manufacturers. The products may be packaged separately or as kits for individuals with incontinence.

Odor Control

The odor associated with urinary incontinence is thought to be due mainly to the production of ammonia from urea by bacterial ureases.[40] If odor is newly evident, it may indicate urinary tract infection; therefore a urine specimen should be sent to the laboratory for culture and sensitivity testing.

To prevent odor, adequate hydration and personal hygiene are essential. Containment products should be changed when they become saturated. If reusable equipment or devices are used, they should be cleansed according to manufacturers' guidelines. The use of external deodorizers may also be of benefit. Orally administered over-the-counter chlorophyll tablets may reduce urinary odor. The deodorizing effect of these tablets is cumulative; up to 7 days of medication may be necessary to reach maximum concentrations. Certain foods, notably asparagus, and specific medications may also cause an unusual odor.

MANAGEMENT OF ENURESIS IN CHILDREN
Definition

Enuresis is defined as nocturnal and diurnal loss of urine in children. Enuresis may be a primary condition, as when a child has never gained control of the bladder, or it may be secondary and occur after a child has been reliably trained for 6 months to 1 year. This discussion is limited to primary, nocturnal, nonorganic (nonpathologic) enuresis, more commonly known as bedwetting. This type of enuresis occurs more often in boys, and the problem tends to be familial.[14]

Enuresis may be recognized when bedwetting occurs after the child has reached a certain age (4, 5, or 6 years) or a particular developmental milestone (for example, when the child starts school). Investigation begins when the bedwetting becomes a concern to the child or parent. The initial workup includes a urinalysis and urine culture, a history and physical, and a stream check. Functional bladder capacity is assessed by measuring the volume of each void for 7 days; the average volume per void is then determined. In obtaining this data it is important not to draw undue attention to the program, since this can skew results. Further studies are indicated only if disease or abnormality is suspected.

Intervention Considerations

If there is no organic cause for the enuresis, the family must decide either to intervene or to wait for spontaneous resolution. Because the incidence of bedwetting decreases from 10% at age 5 and 5% at age 10 to less than 1% at age 18, a "they'll grow out of it" approach is often advocated. However, consideration must be given to the impact of the enuresis on the child's self-esteem and to the social restrictions placed on the child and the family.[14]

With or without intervention, consistent routines must be established. Absorbent products may simplify care, but if the child wakes to void, they are difficult to remove and using them may inhibit motivation by causing the child to feel like an infant.

Responsibility for changing wet sheets must be defined. When changing the sheets is the child's task, it is incorporated into the daily routine and is not a punishment. If parents assume this duty, it is not delegated to the child out of frustration or anger on a "bad morning." All negative feedback connected with the bedwetting must be eliminated.

If the family elects to intervene, it is imperative to enlist the child's full cooperation and participation in the program to maximize the chance of success. The bathroom should have adequate lighting so that the child can easily find it at night. The child should routinely void at bedtime to begin the night with an empty bladder. A sticker chart can be used to record results of the program and provide positive reinforcement.

The two factors most often associated with enuresis are small functional bladder capacity and deep sleep. The child may have one without the other, and interventions for each vary.[14]

Measures to Increase Functional Bladder Capacity

The normal bladder capacity of children who are less than 10 years of age is determined by the following formula: 1 oz per year of age + 1; at 10 years of age the adult capacity is reached. Interventions for expanding bladder capacity include exercise, fluid manipulation, dietary modifications, and medication.

Exercises and Fluid Manipulation. Exercises are performed each time the child feels the urge to void. At the signal to urinate, the child goes to the bathroom and waits for 5 minutes, before emptying the bladder. (Initially the child may not be able to wait for 5 minutes, and it may be necessary to decrease this interval.) When urinating, the child stops the flow in midstream and then starts the stream again. The time intervals and the number of stops and starts are gradually extended according to the age of the child and the child's ability to comply with the program, until normal functional bladder capacity is obtained. The child is encouraged (but not forced) to drink fluids during the day. This practice increases the number of voidings and gives the child more opportunities to exercise. In the evening, fluid intake is limited but not restricted.

Dietary Modifications. Dietary alterations may be helpful. Some children with an allergy to milk will have less enuresis if milk is eliminated from the evening diet. Since salty bedtime snacks increase fluid intake, they are reduced. In addition, the consumption of foods and fluids with a diuretic effect (for example, sodas, caffeinated drinks, and chocolate) should be discouraged.[49]

Pharmacologic Manipulation. Medications may be used to reduce bladder contractility and thereby improve functional bladder capacity (Table 4-2). Use of medications is controversial; some pediatricians think the use of medications is inappropriate in the case of a "benign" condition such as bedwetting; other physicians think the use of medications is appropriate for selected patients during a specific time. Side effects of medications include dry mouth, blurred vision, and constipation. Two to 3 months after the desired effect is obtained, medication dosages should be tapered to prevent "rebound enuresis." Diuretics are not used in treatment, although they may be recommended on special occasions to allow a child to participate in overnight activities.[14]

Table 4-2 Medications used in treatment of enuresis

Category	Generic name	Action
Antispasmodic	Oxybutynin	Reduces uninhibited bladder contractions
Anticholinergic	Imipramine	Reduces uninhibited bladder contractions
Antidepressant	Imipramine	Decreases depth of sleep
Antidiuretic	Desmopressin	Induces temporary water retention
Diuretic		Induces moderate dehydration

Interventions for Deep Sleep

Some children sleep through the signal of bladder fullness. Interventions for deep sleep include waking and medication.

Methods for Waking. Waking can be accomplished in four different ways. The child *must* be thoroughly awake before toileting. The easiest method of waking is a simple form of self-hypnosis, or visualization. Each night on going to bed, the child mentally images waking at the sense of a full bladder, stopping the flow of urine, getting up, finding the bathroom, voiding into the toilet, and returning to a dry bed. Another method of waking is the use of an alarm system. These systems are compact, lightweight, battery operated, and easy to assemble. A sensor is attached to the child's underwear and connected to a buzzer that is worn on the collar or wrist. The alarm is activated by a few drops of urine and wakes the child, triggering contraction of the external sphincter. This conditions the child to wake at the sensation of bladder distention. These devices work better for older children who can be independently responsible for using them. An alarm clock can be used to wake the child at gradually increasing time intervals, or the parent can wake and toilet the child during the night. However, since these methods involve arbitrary timings not associated with bladder fullness, they may be less effective.[14]

Pharmacologic Manipulation. Medications (for example, imipramine) can be used to decrease the depth of sleep. In addition to reducing the depth of the child's sleep, imipramine has an anticholinergic effect, which may improve bladder capacity. Side effects (dry mouth, blurred vision, and constipation) and cases of overdose, one resulting in death, have been reported. Two to 3 months after the desired effect is obtained, dosages should be tapered to reduce the risk of relapse. Children who relapse when use of the drug is discontinued may not respond to subsequent courses of treatment.

Recently enuresis has been associated with a lack of antidiuretic hormone during the night, and titrated doses of 1-deamino-8-D-arginine vasopressin (DDAVP) have been recommended. This treatment is expensive; the cost currently ranges from $125 to $250 per month.[45]

The parents and child need support throughout the intervention period. Small successes are often overlooked; the nurse must point these out to the family and stress that progress is gradual. If the child loses interest, it may be necessary to suggest stopping the program temporarily.

SUMMARY

The goals in the management of urinary incontinence are (1) to restore continence or establish a plan for incontinence management that enables the patient to maintain or resume his or her life-style and (2) to prevent deterioration of the upper urinary tract. The nurse's role is to devise, in collaboration with the patient and the health care team, a bladder management program that accomplishes these goals and is both manageable by and acceptable to the patient and family.

SELF-EVALUATION

QUESTIONS

1. Identify the two major goals in the management of patients with urinary incontinence.
2. Identify commonly used treatments for the following types of incontinence:
   a. Stress incontinence
   b. Instability (urge) incontinence
   c. Instability (reflex) incontinence
   d. Overflow incontinence (urinary retention)
   e. Continual (extraurethral or total) incontinence
3. Identify functional factors that should be assessed and addressed for all patients who have incontinence.
4. Identify the muscles that are exercised in a program of pelvic floor exercises, and identify two approaches to teaching patients how to isolate these muscles.
5. Explain why a pessary device may decrease stress incontinence and when such a device is indicated.
6. Differentiate a prompted voiding program from a bladder drill program.
7. Identify measures used to increase functional bladder capacity.
8. The treatment of choice for most patients with reflex incontinence and bladder-sphincter dyssynergia is:
   a. Clean intermittent catheterization with or without anticholinergics
   b. Indwelling catheter
   c. Bladder drill program
   d. Sympathomimetic drugs and prompted voiding
9. Identify patients who may benefit from each of the following:
   a. Sympathomimetic drugs (alpha-adrenergic agonists)
   b. Anticholinergics and smooth-muscle relaxants
   c. Alpha-adrenergic blocking agents
   d. Conjugated estrogens
10. Identify key areas to be addressed in teaching patients the procedure for clean intermittent catheterization.
11. Explain why medical or surgical sphincterotomy is frequently required for men with reflex incontinence that is being managed with condom drainage.
12. Significant urinary tract infection (in contrast to simple bacteriuria) is likely to be characterized by:
    a. Suprapubic discomfort or flank discomfort, fever, and nausea
    b. Cloudy, malodorous urine and increased sediment in the urine
    c. Slight leakage around the catheter and bloody urine

13. Identify the goal of surgical intervention for the patient with stress incontinence related to pelvic floor relaxation, and identify at least one surgical option for this patient.

14. Explain the goal of surgical intervention for the patient with stress incontinence related to intrinsic sphincter dysfunction, and identify at least two surgical options for this patient.

15. Identify the three components of the artificial urinary sphincter.

16. Which of the following most frequently necessitates the removal of an artificial urinary sphincter?
    a. Pressure necrosis and ulceration
    b. Infection and erosion
    c. Tissue trauma and hemorrhage
    d. Total urethral obstruction

17. Which of the following patients is likely to benefit from augmentation cystoplasty?
    a. Patient with stress incontinence
    b. Patient with overflow incontinence
    c. Patient with functional incontinence
    d. Patient with instability incontinence (urge or reflex)

18. Identify the primary effect of each of the following on bladder-sphincter function:
    a. Anticholinergic drugs
    b. Smooth-muscle relaxants
    c. Alpha-adrenergic agonists
    d. Conjugated estrogens
    e. Cholinergic agents
    f. Alpha-adrenergic blocking agents

19. Identify at least two criteria for effective use of external (condom) catheters for men.

20. Identify at least two situations in which the use of indwelling catheters is appropriate.

21. True or False: A urine culture and sensitivity test should be performed for the patient with an indwelling catheter at least monthly so that bacteriuria can be treated promptly.

22. Identify two types of absorbent products for ambulatory patients.

23. Identify two types of products used to provide skin protection for the patient with continual incontinence.

24. Identify the two factors thought to contribute to enuresis.

25. Identify one treatment for each of the causative factors in enuresis.

SELF-EVALUATION

ANSWERS

1. **a.** Restore continence or develop an acceptable bladder management program.
   b. Protect the function of the upper urinary tract (kidneys)
2. **a.** Stress incontinence
      Pelvic floor exercises
      Sympathomimetic (alpha-adrenergic) drugs
      Pessary placement
      Surgical intervention (to correct altered urethrovesical anatomy or improve urethral resistance)
   b. Instability (urge) incontinence
      Toileting programs (prompted voiding program or bladder drill program)
      Anticholinergics and smooth-muscle relaxants
      Environmental modifications
      Elimination of bladder irritants
      Biofeedback and pelvic floor exercises
   c. Instability (reflex) incontinence
      Clean intermittent catheterization with pharmacologic manipulation (anticholinergics)
      Reflex voiding with condom drainage
   d. Overflow incontinence (urinary retention)
      Double voiding and fluid control programs
      Alpha-adrenergic blocking agents
      Clean intermittent catheterization
      Indwelling catheter
   e. Continual (extraurethral or total) incontinence
      Correction of underlying cause
      Containment and skin care
3. **a.** Mobility and access deficits
   b. Dexterity deficits
   c. Deficits of mentation and motivation
4. Periurethral muscles. (1) Biofeedback. Simultaneous tracings of periurethral muscle contractions and abdominal muscle contractions help the patient learn to contract the right muscle. (2) The examiner places a gloved finger into the patient's vaginal vault or anal canal and provides the patient with verbal feedback while the patient is learning to contract the correct muscles.

5. A pessary device improves sphincter function by restoring more normal urethral position. Such a device is indicated for the patient who is not a surgical candidate and who does not respond to exercise programs.

6. **a.** A prompted voiding program establishes a fixed schedule for voiding based on the results of a voiding diary. The intent of the program is to teach the patient to voluntarily initiate voiding before the bladder gets full enough to cause leakage.

   b. A bladder drill program establishes a strict voiding schedule, and the interval between voidings is gradually increased. The intent of the program is to teach the patient to inhibit bladder contractions and increase functional bladder capacity. Patients participating in these programs need intensive support.

7. **a.** Anticholinergics and smooth-muscle relaxants
   b. Augmentation cystoplasty
   c. Bladder drill programs

8. **a.** Clean intermittent catheterization with or without anticholinergics.

9. **a.** Sympathomimetic drugs: patient with stress incontinence
   b. Anticholinergics and smooth-muscle relaxants: patient with bladder instability (urge or reflex incontinence)
   c. Alpha-adrenergic blocking agents: patient with DESD

10. Positioning for perineal access
    Aseptic technique (clean, dry hands and clean, lubricated catheter)
    Location of the urethral meatus
    Technique for insertion of the catheter
    Care and transport of catheters
    Recognition and management of infection

11. Most patients with reflex voiding also have bladder-sphincter dyssynergia as a result of a suprasacral lesion that interrupts the pontine-sacral axis.

12. Suprapubic discomfort or flank discomfort, fever, and nausea

13. To restore the bladder neck and urethra to intra-abdominal position. Surgical interventions include anterior urethropexy and modified Pereyra bladder neck suspension.

14. To increase urethral resistance by providing urethral compression. Surgical interventions include the pubovaginal sling procedure, periurethral injections of collagen or Teflon, and the artificial urinary sphincter implant.

15. The urethral cuff, the pressure-regulating balloon, and the control pump

16. **b.** Infection and erosion

17. **d.** Patient with instability incontinence (urge or reflex)

18. **a.** Anticholinergic drugs
       Reduce bladder contractility
       Increase functional capacity.

    b. Smooth-muscle relaxants

        Reduce bladder contractility

        Increase functional bladder capacity

    c. Alpha-adrenergic agonists

        Increase urethral resistance

    d. Conjugated estrogens

        Stimulate proliferation of urethral mucosa, thereby increasing urethral resistance (for patients with estrogen deficiency and atrophic vaginitis)

    e. Cholinergic agents

        Increase bladder contractility

    f. Alpha-adrenergic blocking agents

        Decrease urethral resistance

19. a. Appropriate sizing and fit of the catheter

    b. Adequate adherence of the sheath of the catheter to the penile skin

    c. Molding at the connecting end of the catheter, which prevents twisting

20. a. A case of overflow incontinence associated with unresectable obstruction

    b. Instances in which the patient or family members or both decide that dryness and comfort outweigh the risks of using an indwelling catheter (for example, a patient with a terminal illness).

    c. A situation in which urinary incontinence is impeding the healing of a wound or threatening the integrity of the skin.

    d. A case in which pain severely limits the patient's ability to complete toileting and change garments.

21. False

22. Inserts, pads with straps, and pad-and-pants systems

23. Skin sealants (copolymer films) and moisture barrier ointments

24. a. Reduced functional bladder capacity

    b. Deep sleep

25. a. Sphincter exercises, fluid control, and dietary alterations

    b. Waking methods and medications

REFERENCES

1. Alvaro J and Gartley W: Products and devices for managing incontinence. In Gartley C, ed: Managing incontinence: a guide to living with loss of bladder control, Ottawa, Ill, 1985, Jameson Books, Inc.
2. Andersson KE: Current concepts in the treatment of disorders of micturition, Drugs 35:477, 1988.
3. Barrett DM and Wein AJ: Adult and pediatric urology, vol 1, Chicago, 1987, Mosby–Year Book, Inc.
4. Baum M: Urinary incontinence, Crit Care Update 9[11]: 27, 1982.
5. Brink CA and Wells TJ: Environmental support for geriatric incontinence: toilets, toilet supplements, and external equipment, Clin Geriatr Med 2[4]:829, 1986.
6. Cardozo LD and Stanton SL: Biofeedback: a five year review, Br J Urol 56:220, 1985.
7. Cottenden AM: Incontinence pads and appliances, Int Disabil Stud 10[1]:44, 1988.
8. Dougherty MC, Abrams RA, and McKey PA: An instrument to assess the dynamic characteristics of the circumvaginal musculature, Nurs Res 35:202, 1985.
9. Dougherty MC et al: The effect of exercise on the circumvaginal muscles in postpartum women, J Nurse Midwifery 34:8, 1989.
10. Douglas C et al: Microwave: practical, cost-effective method for sterilizing urinary catheters in the home, Urology 35:219, 1990.
11. Duckett JW and Snyder HM: Continent urinary diversion: variations on the Mitrofanoff principle, J Urol 136:58, 1986.
12. Duffin HM and Castledon CM: The continence nurse adviser's role in the British health care system, Clin Geriatr Med 2[4]:841, 1986.
13. Eriksen BC, Bergmann S, and Eik-Nes SH: Maximal electrostimulation of the pelvic floor in female idiopathic detrusor instability and urge incontinence, Neurourol Urodyn 8:219, 1989.
14. Faller NA: Enuresis, J Enterost Ther 14[2]:66, 1987.
15. Faller NA and Vinson RK: The artificial urinary sphincter, J Enterost Ther 12[1]:7, 1985.
16. Fantl JA et al: Bladder training in community dwelling women with urinary incontinence, Abstract from the Consensus Development Conference: Urinary incontinence in adults, Bethesda, Md, 1988.
17. Feneley RCL: The management of female incontinence by suprapubic catheterization, with or without urethral closure, Br J Urol 55:203, 1983.
18. Fishman IJ, Shabsigh R and Scott FB: Experience with the artificial urinary sphincter model AS800 in 148 patients, J Urol 141:307, 1989.
19. Freiha FS and Stamey TA: Cystolysis: a procedure for the selective denervation of the bladder, J Urol 123:360, 1980.
20. Goldwasser B, Furlow WL, and Barrett D: The model AMS800 artificial urinary sphincter: Mayo Clinic experience, J Urol 137:668, 1987.
21. Govoni LE and Hayes JE: Drugs and nursing implications, Norwalk, CT, 1982, Appleton-Century-Croft.
22. Gray ML: Functional incontinence. In Thompson JM et al, eds: Clinical nursing, ed 2, St Louis, 1989, Mosby–Year Book, Inc.
23. Gray ML and Dobkin KA: Genitourinary system. In Thompson JM et al, eds: Clinical nursing, ed 2, St Louis, 1989, Mosby–Year Book, Inc.
24. Hagen B et al: The effects of two different pelvic floor muscle exercise programs in treatment of urinary stress incontinence in women, Neurourol Urodyn 8[Abstract 43], 1989.
25. Hollister, Inc: Female urinary pouch clinical report, Project 232, Libertyville, Ill, 1986, Hollister, Inc.
26. Jagachandran S, Moopphan U, and Kim H: Complications from external (condom) urinary drainage devices, Urology 25[1]:31, 1985.
27. Jarvis GJ: A controlled trial of bladder drill and drug therapy in the management of detrusor instability, Br J Urol 53:565, 1981.
28. Kaufman M et al: Transurethral polytetrafluoroethylene injection for post prostatectomy urinary incontinence, J Urol 132:463, 1984.

29. Kegel AH: Progressive resistance exercise in the functional restoration of the perineal muscles, Am J Obstet Gynecol 56:238, 1948.
30. Kim MJ, McFarland GH, and McLane AM: Pocket guide to nursing diagnoses, ed 3, St Louis, 1989, Mosby–Year Book, Inc.
31. King A: Nursing management of stomas of the genitourinary system. In Broadwell DC and Jackson BJ, eds: Principles of ostomy care, St Louis, 1982, Mosby–Year Book, Inc.
32. Kniep-Hardy MJ, Votava K, and Stubbings MJ: Managing indwelling catheters in the home, Geriatr Nurs 6[5]:280, 1985.
33. Kock NG et al: Urinary diversion via a continent ileal reservoir: clinical results in 12 patients, J Urol 128:469, 1982.
34. Lapides J et al: Further observations on self catheterization, Trans Am Assoc Genito-Urinary Surgeons 67:15, 1975.
35. Leach GE, O'Donnell P, and Raz S: Needle urethral-vesical suspension procedures. In Raz S, ed: Female urology, Philadelphia, 1983, WB Saunders Co.
36. Linder A, Leach GE, and Raz S: Augmentation cystoplasty in the treatment of neurogenic bladder dysfunction. J Urol 129:491, 1983.
37. Lindstrom S et al: The neurophysiological basis of bladder inhibition in response to intravaginal electrical stimulation, J Urol 129:405, 1983.
38. McCormick KA, Scheve AAS, and Leahy E: Nursing management of urinary incontinence in geriatric inpatients, Nurs Clin North Am 23[1]:231, 1988.
39. McGuire EJ and Lytton B: Pubovaginal sling procedure for stress incontinence, J Urol 119:82, 1978.
40. Norberg A et al: The urine smell around patients with urinary incontinence: the production of ammonia in ordinary diapers and in diapers impregnated with copper acetate, Gerontology 30:261, 1984.
41. Olin BR: Professional's guide to patient drug facts, ed 1, Philadelphia, 1990, JB Lippincott Co.
42. Politano VA: Periurethral polytetrafluoroethylene injection for urinary incontinence, J Urol 127:439, 1982.
43. Regensberg D: Objective: social continence, catheter challenges, Nursing RSA Verpleging 2[4]:16, 1987.
44. Resnick N and Subbarao YV: Management of urinary incontinence in the elderly, N Engl J Med 313[13]:800, 1985.
45. Rittig S et al: Long range double blind cross over study of DDAVP intranasal spray in the management of nocturnal enuresis, Neurourol Urodyn 7[3]:184, 1988.
46. Roe BH and Brocklehurst JC: Patients' perceptions of their catheters, Neurourol Urodyn 6 [Abstract 29], 1987.
47. Romanowski GL et al: Urinary incontinence in the elderly: etiology and treatment, Drug Intell Clin Pharm 22:525, 1988.
48. Rowland RG et al: Indiana continent urinary reservoir, J Urol 137:1136, 1987.
49. Scharf MB: Waking up dry: how to end bedwetting forever, Cincinnati, 1986, Writer's Digest Books.
50. Scott FB: The use of the artificial sphincter in the treatment of urinary incontinence in the female patient, Urol Clin North Am 12:305, 1985.
51. Scott FB: The artificial urinary sphincter: experience in adults, Urol Clin North Am 16[1]:105, 1989.
52. Shortliffe LMD et al: Treatment of urinary incontinence by the periurethral implantation of glutaraldehyde linked collagen, J Urol 141:538, 1989.
53. Siegel SW and Montague DK: Surgery for stress urinary incontinence. In Stewart's operative urology, ed 2, vol 2, Baltimore, 1989, Williams & Wilkins.
54. Skidmore-Roth L: Mosby's 1990 nursing drug reference, St Louis, 1990, Mosby–Year Book, Inc.
55. Spencer JR, O'Conor VJ, and Schaeffer A: A comparison of endoscopic suspension of the vesical neck with suprapubic vesicourethropexy for treatment of stress urinary incontinence, J Urol 137:411, 1987.

56. Stanton SL: Vaginal prolapse, In Raz S, ed: Female urology, Philadelphia, 1983, WB Saunders Co.

57. Staskin DR et al: The pathophysiology of stress incontinence, Urol Clin North Am 12:271, 1985.

58. Tanagho EA, Schmidt RA, and Orvis BR: Neural stimulation for control of voiding dysfunction: preliminary report in 22 patients with serious neuropathic voiding disorders, J Urol 142:340, 1989.

59. Tovell H and Danforth D: Structural defects and relaxations. In Danforth D and Scott J, eds: Obstetrics and gynecology, ed 5, Philadelphia, 1986, JB Lippincott Co.

60. Warren J: Catheters and catheter care, Clin Geriatr Med 2[4]:857, 1986.

61. Weiss B: Chronic indwelling bladder catheterization, Am Fam Physician 30[3]:161, 1984.

62. White H: Aids to continence: simple and sophisticated, Medical Education [International] Ltd: Nursing [Oxford] 2[29]:855, 1984.

5 Continence Clinics

ELLEN SHIPES

OBJECTIVES

1. Identify the three phases in the process of establishing a continence clinic.
2. Explain the significance of marketing research in determining the need for a continence clinic.
3. Identify the resources that must be allocated before a continence clinic can be established.
4. Identify the functions of a continence clinic, including direct and indirect services.
5. List the major target groups and promotional strategies to be considered in a marketing plan.
6. Identify resources for patients and professionals who deal with incontinence.

In this chapter the development of continence clinics and support groups for the management of urinary incontinence is discussed. The term "continence clinic" has been chosen deliberately to avoid the negative connotations of the term "incontinence clinic."

Urinary incontinence is a major problem for both the health care community and the public.[2,4,5] In response, more and more continence clinics and support groups are being developed. A well-planned, well-coordinated continence clinic provides comprehensive diagnosis, treatment, and follow-up care in the community setting. Continence clinics may be operated full time or part time; they may be incorporated within an existing facility or free standing.

ESTABLISHED CLINICS

Many continence clinics already exist in the United States, and their number is growing rapidly. Information about these clinics may be obtained from the organizations listed in the box below; urologists may also be sources of information.

PROCESS FOR ESTABLISHING A CONTINENCE CLINIC

The viability and efficacy of a continence clinic depends on extensive planning and development. Specific, concrete actions can be taken to increase the prospect of success. Gross and Bailey provided a wealth of information about establishing clinics; although their work was addressed to enterostomal therapy (ET) nurses, the material they presented is extensive and can be applied to any clinic.[3]

Brink, Wells, and Diokno have identified three phases in the process of establishing a continence clinic: development, operation, and evaluation.[1] The development phase is extensive and includes the following components: assessment of need, identification and allocation of resources, establishment of organizational and functional activities, and marketing. Operation and evaluation proceed naturally from the plan for development. In the following section each aspect of development is discussed in detail.

ORGANIZATIONS THAT PROVIDE INFORMATION ABOUT ESTABLISHED CONTINENCE CLINICS

Help for Incontinent People (HIP)
P.O. Box 544
Union, SC 29379

Incontinence Treatment Center
Presbyterian Medical Center of Philadelphia
39th and Market Street
Philadelphia, PA 19104

Simon Foundation, Inc.
Box 815
Wilmette, IL 60091

Development

Assessment of Need. The first and most important aspect of development is to determine the need for a continence clinic. Market research should provide clear, concise information about the need for a clinic. Studies of demographic data, the proximity of similar services, and the availability of referral sources should be included in this research.

In obtaining demographic data, the researcher evaluates the population in the area for characteristics associated with a problem or condition; when incontinence is being studied, the characteristics of age, sex, multiparity, diabetes, birth defects, and handicaps are evaluated. The number of retirement centers and long-term care facilities in the community must also be determined. Sources of data include public libraries, demographic record departments of regional courthouses, district health centers, area agencies on aging, and social service departments. Additional resources include health clinics, geriatric centers, the American Cancer Society, the United Ostomy Association, and health care professionals. A direct-mail questionnaire that may be answered anonymously can be sent to community health care consumers in general or can be targeted to specific populations such as residents of senior citizen centers and retirement centers or those who seek medical advice at women's health centers. Fig. 5-1 illustrates an anonymously answered direct-mail questionnaire. Data obtained from the questionnaire can be extrapolated to the general population and may provide information about the types and severity of incontinence in the population, treatment being provided, and the population's knowledge and use of resources. It is often cost effective to hire a professional research firm to obtain this demographic data and to present it in a form that supports the need for a continence clinic.

Since competition for services can be detrimental to the success of a clinic, the proximity of other clinics such as women's health centers or urology clinics that offer similar services must be assessed. The local medical referral service and the Yellow Pages of the local phone book are sources of data concerning the proximity of similar services.

Proposal. The next step in the development phase is to write a proposal. The proposal should include a statement of the purpose, goals, and objectives of the continence clinic.

Identification and Allocation of Resources. The success of a clinic depends on the quality and quantity of the clinic's resources. These resources include the physical plant, equipment, personnel, funding, and referrals.[3]

Physical plant. The clinic itself comprises the physical plant. It should be in a readily accessible location and provide full access to individuals with handicaps, and parking should be inexpensive or free. The size of clinics varies, but

Date of birth _____ Age _____ Sex Male _____ Female _____

Women only   **Men only**

Number of children   1-2 _____   Prostate problems   Yes _____ No _____
                      3-5 _____
                      5-7 _____   Prostate operation   Yes _____ No _____
                      7+ _____
Difficult deliveries
Yes _____ No _____

Urinary history

Bladder infection   Yes _____ No _____
Urinary operation   Yes _____ No _____
Kidney infection   Yes _____ No _____
Operation on reproductive organs   Yes _____ No _____

Urinary symptoms

Frequent voiding (every 1 to 2 hours)   Yes _____ No _____
Urge to void   Yes _____ No _____
Warning time _____
Voiding at night   Yes _____ No _____
Number of times _____
Straining to void   Yes _____ No _____
Pain on voiding   Yes _____ No _____
Dribbling urine   Yes _____ No _____
Stress incontinence   Yes _____ No _____
  (leak during cough, sneeze, etc.)
Hesitancy (takes time to start)   Yes _____ No _____
Blood in urine   Yes _____ No _____

Are you incontinent now?   Yes _____ No _____
Have you had treatment?   Yes _____ No _____
Are you currently taking medicine?   Yes _____ No _____
Surgery?   Yes _____ No _____

Other _____

Did treatment help?   Yes _____ No _____
Does incontinence limit your life-style? Yes _____ No _____
Is incontinence a minor problem?   Yes _____ No _____
Is incontinence a major problem?   Yes _____ No _____

Fig. 5-1   Direct-mail questionnaire, which may be used to determine need for continence clinic.

the physical plant should be large enough to provide all the necessary services without crowding. Minimum requirements are (1) a waiting room and registration area, (2) an examining room, (3) a room for diagnosis and treatment, (4) an office, and (5) a bathroom. Clinics associated with a larger institution use the laboratory and radiology services of that institution; free-standing clinics must provide these services in some way that is convenient to daily operation. Providing these resources on a contractual basis may be cost effective.

Equipment. To offer the best care, a full-service clinic must have state-of-the-art equipment. Necessary equipment includes diagnostic equipment (for example, urodynamic testing equipment), equipment for treatment (for example, biofeedback equipment), equipment for the examining room (for example, an examining table, storage for supplies, and a well-lighted area for examination and teaching), office equipment (for example, files, chairs, and desks), and miscellaneous equipment (such as linens). Equipment recommended for continence clinics is listed in the box below.

Personnel. A sufficient number of experienced personnel is vital to the clinic's success. The number of personnel depends on the size of the clinic and the

---

EQUIPMENT RECOMMENDED FOR A CONTINENCE CLINIC

DIAGNOSTIC EQUIPMENT
Urodynamics
Laboratory
Radiology

EXAMINING ROOM EQUIPMENT
Table and step stool
Light source
Equipment and supply table
Storage area
Writing table
Three chairs (minimum)
Sink
Disposable supplies (for example,
   catheterization supplies, specimen
   containers, underpads, inconti-
   nence products, examining room
   supplies)
Wastebaskets
Linen
Patient education information
Mirror (hand mirror or full-length
   mirror or both)

TREATMENT EQUIPMENT
Biofeedback
Pelvic floor stimulation
Clean intermittent catheterization
Containment devices and skin care
   products

OFFICE EQUIPMENT
Desk and chair for each person
Typewriter and computer
Storage for supplies
File cabinets
Two additional chairs (minimum)
Telephone
Office supplies

projected number of clients. Initially personnel may be shared with another institution. The minimum number of personnel includes a medical director (a urologist or an internist with a background in geriatrics), a program manager (a urology nurse, an ET nurse, or another nurse knowledgeable in the management of incontinence), a nurse or a technician skilled in performing and interpreting urodynamic and biofeedback testing, and a secretary or receptionist or both. Larger clinics may include additional staff (for example, a urologist, a gynecologist, a behavioral therapist, or a combination of these). Ancillary staff include laboratory and radiology technicians and marketing, financial, legal, supply, transportation, and housekeeping personnel. Some of these staff members work for the clinic as consultants or work part time.

Funding and allocation of funds. Funds should be adequate to purchase necessary supplies and equipment and to pay for salaries, rent, utilities, repairs, maintenance, travel and education, marketing, and dues and subscriptions until the clinic becomes self-sustaining, which takes approximately 2 years. Funds may be available from several sources, such as the parent institution, physicians, grants, state vocational rehabilitation programs, consultation and lecture fees, and patient charges.[3]

Patient charges are generated from visits, surgery, biofeedback therapy, diagnostic tests, teaching, and supplies. Charging mechanisms vary, but usually the patient is charged a flat fee for each clinic visit and diagnostic study; additional charges for supplies vary. Amounts charged should be competitive with fees for similar services within the community.

Referrals. Each clinic must determine its own referral policy. Many clinics accept self-referrals, as well as referrals from such health care professionals as physicians, nurses, social workers, and pharmacists.

Establishment of Organizational and Functional Activities. An organizational chart establishes a clear, concrete chain of command (Fig. 5-2). Organizational structure facilitates communication throughout the chain and optimizes clinic functions. Vital to organizational strength are job descriptions, policies, and procedures.

Job descriptions detail roles and responsibilities of each staff member. Well-written job descriptions set forth educational and experiential requirements specific to each position. Expectations should be clear and agreeable to both employer and employee.

Policies are facility-determined, written guidelines that direct the management of the clinic. Procedures provide standards and guidelines for services provided. Record forms and record keeping, along with attention to budgetary needs, are significant components in organizational operation.

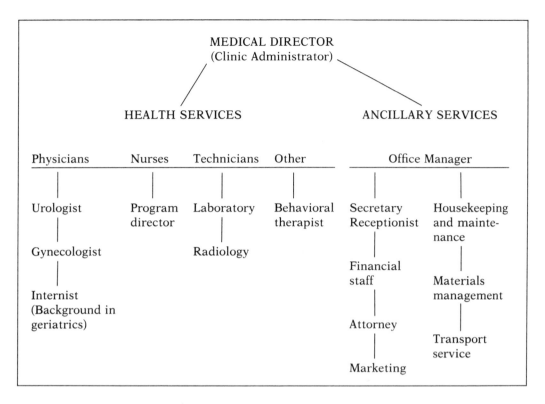

Fig. 5-2 Suggested organizational structure for continence clinic. Number of personnel is based on size of clinic and projected number of patients. Positions vary according to needs of individual clinics.

Function. Clinic functions are the services provided by the clinic and are tailored to meet the needs of both the clinic and the patients. Clinic services can be direct or indirect. Direct services include assessment, diagnosis, treatment, and follow-up. Indirect services include patient, family, and community education and such support services as social services and transportation.

Direct services

ASSESSMENT

Assessment often begins 1 week before the first clinic visit. The patient may be asked to keep a voiding diary that records the time of voiding, the amount of urine voided, any feeling of urgency, and incontinent episodes. On admission to the clinic the patient is usually assessed by the nurse program manager or the ET nurse. The nurse conducts a thorough assessment, which includes the general reason for the visit, the patient's general physical and emotional status,

Date _____

Name _____   Age _____   Date of birth _____

Address _____   Sex   Male _____   Female _____

Physician _____

Referred by _____

Reason for visit _____

_____

Urinary symptoms

Frequency _____
Nocturia _____   Times per night _____
Urgency _____
Stress _____
Enuresis _____   Times per week _____

_____

Voiding symptoms

Hesitancy _____
Straining _____
Dysuria _____
Hematuria   Initial _____   Continuous _____   End _____
Change in stream _____
Dribbling   Occasional _____   Continuous _____

Incontinence

When it began _____
Changes   Better _____   Worse _____   No change _____
Frequency (times per day) _____
Previous treatments _____
Effectiveness of treatments _____
Incontinence aids used   Type _____   Times per day _____   Effectiveness _____

_____

Medical history

Previous illnesses and operations _____
Number of pregnancies _____   Any difficulty? _____
Current medications _____

_____

Fig. 5-3   Admission assessment form. (Adapted from Jeter K, Faller N, and Norton C, eds: Nursing for continence, Philadelphia, 1990, WB Saunders.)

General health

Bowel habits   Constipation _____   Laxatives _____
Systemic disease   Diabetes _____   Heart problems _____
                            Arthritis _____
Vision _____
Dexterity _____
Foot problems _____
Mobility _____   Aids used _____

Environment

Location of toilet _____
Number of people sharing toilet _____
Aids for toileting _____
Lighting in bathroom _____

Emotional health

Attitude toward incontinence _____

Impact of incontinence on life-style _____

Attitude of others in family _____

Anxiety _____   Depression _____   Hopelessness _____   Other _____
Intact mental abilities? _____

Support systems

Live with _____
Visitors _____
Social activities   Church _____   Shopping _____   Visting _____   Other_____
Altered relationships due to incontinence _____
Community services used _____

Results of physical examination

Rectal examination _____
Vaginal examination _____
Skin problems _____   Other_____

Goals _____

Action plan _____

socioeconomic background, and perception of incontinence, the impact of incontinence on the patient's life-style, previous treatments and results, and the patient's medical history, living environment, support system, and expectations about clinic interventions (Fig. 5-3).

DIAGNOSIS

The physician determines the diagnosis based on the results of a thorough history and physical examination and diagnostic tests. The diagnosis is discussed with the patient and family, and time is provided for questions and answers.

TREATMENT

Selection of a treatment plan is collaborative, involving the treatment team and the patient, and is based on the results of the diagnostic workup. Treatment options include surgery, medications, biofeedback, toileting programs, clean intermittent catheterization, pelvic floor exercises, environmental modifications, the selection of appropriate containment devices, and skin care. Patient and family counseling and education are key to all treatment plans. The nurse plays a vital role in comprehensive assessment and in patient education and counseling; in some settings the nurse also administers diagnostic tests and biofeedback therapy.

FOLLOW-UP CARE

Follow-up care is essential for all patients. Many clinics routinely schedule three visits: the first for assessment and testing, the second for treatment and counseling, and the third for follow-up care and continued teaching. Patients or caregivers should be contacted and reminded of follow-up visits, and additional visits can be scheduled as necessary.

Indirect services

SOCIAL SERVICES

Social services are essential in assisting patients and families with the many financial concerns related to seeking and continuing successful treatment for incontinence.

TRANSPORTATION

In some sections of the country, assistance with transportation contributes heavily to the success of the clinic. Some clinics provide vans to transport patients to and from the clinic. This service is vital in areas where many patients are elderly, ill, or poor. In such areas lack of transportation can be an impediment to treatment.

Promotional Activities. A well-developed, well-coordinated, properly inaugurated marketing plan is essential to the clinic's success. An important component of marketing is promotion of services to appropriate target groups. Promotion can be quite innovative and should employ all forms of media for the greatest effect. Promotion can be as extravagant as advertising the clinic's services in a widely distributed city newspaper or on television, or as simple

---

PROMOTIONAL STRATEGIES

I. Target groups
  A. Health care industry
    1. Physicians*
      a. Urologists
      b. Gynecologists
      c. Geriatricians
      d. Internists
    2. Nurses
      a. Home care
      b. Discharge planning
      c. Long-term care
      d. Rehabilitation
      e. Geriatrics
      f. Urology
    3. Durable medical equipment dealers
    4. Health maintenance organizations
  B. Community
    1. Senior citizen's programs
    2. Retirement centers
    3. Churches
    4. Community organizations (for example, Kiwanis Club, Lion's Club, American Business Women's Association)

II. Promotional techniques
  A. Media
    1. TV ads during local health-related programs
    2. Radio ads during local health programs
    3. Ads in local or regional newspapers
    4. Senior citizens' newsletters
    5. Health columns in newspapers
  B. Mail campaigns
    1. Letters to physicians (to seek referrals and explain purpose of clinic)
    2. Letters to target audiences
  C. Presentations and seminars
  D. Other techniques
    1. Ads in physicians' newsletters
    2. Networking
    3. Medical resource information services (such as Ask-a-Nurse)
    4. Flyers (posted at supermarkets, durable medical equipment dealers, physicians' offices, churches, pharmacies, and laundromats)
    5. Health fairs

---

*Fig. 5-4 illustrates a sample letter to a physician.

as posting flyers on bulletin boards at senior citizens' centers. The box above outlines other promotional strategies.

Evaluation

Quality assurance activities are an important evaluation tool. When the clinic's success is being evaluated, the following data should be considered: the number of patients, the types of treatment, outcomes of treatments, the number of professional referrals, and patient satisfaction.[1] These types of data should

September 10, 1990

1234 Main St.
Anywhere, USA 12345

John Doe, MD
2468 21st Ave., Suite 246
Anywhere, USA 12345

Dear Dr. Doe,

As you know, urinary incontinence is a problem for many people in our community. Because of your interest in and concern for total health care, we are pleased to inform you of a new service that you might find beneficial for a number of your patients.

We are excited to announce that on October 15, 1990, we will be initiating the services of the Community Continence Clinic at 1234 Main St. Services of the clinic include assessment, diagnosis, and treatment of all types of urinary incontinence. We invite you to visit the Community Continence Clinic at your earliest convenience.

We look forward to working with you in providing specialized care for this particular group of patients with unique needs. Enclosed you will find a brochure that details our services and hours of operation.

Please feel free to call us for further information.

Sincerely,

James Smith, MD
Clinic Director

Joan James, RN MSN CETN
Clinic Manager

Fig. 5-4   Sample letter to physician.

be tabulated routinely, discussed with the program managers, and incorporated into promotional materials.

SUPPORT GROUPS

A continence clinic that offers a support group provides an important component of each patient's bladder management program and a valuable service to the community. Support groups help patients and families to adjust to the feelings associated with incontinence and to discover healthy ways to understand, share, and cope with these feelings. In addition, support groups serve as forums for continuing education. There are both national and local support groups. National groups serve as clearinghouses for education and information about incontinence and related products and may be involved in regulatory activities aimed at improving compensation for incontinence-related interventions and products. Some national groups also assist in the development of local support groups. Prominent support groups are listed in the box below.

PROFESSIONAL ORGANIZATIONS

Several associations for health care professionals are excellent sources of information about incontinence, including the names and locations of practitioners interested in incontinence and its management. These associations are listed in the box on p. 164.

SUPPORT GROUPS

Association of Continence Advisors
c/o Disabled Living Foundation
380-384 Harrows Road
London W92HC, England

Continence Restored, Inc.
785 Park Avenue
New York, NY 10021

Help for Incontinent People (HIP)
P.O. Box 544
Union, SC 29379

International Continence Society
11 West Graham Street
Glasgow G4 9LF, Scotland

Simon Foundation, Inc.
Box 815
Wilmette, IL 60091

ASSOCIATIONS FOR HEALTH CARE PROFESSIONALS

International Association for Enterostomal Therapy (IAET)
2081 Business Center Drive, Suite 290
Irvine, CA 92715-1117
(714) 476-0268

American Urological Association, Allied (AUAA)
6845 Lake Shore Drive (P.O. Box 9397)
Raytown, MO 64133

Association of Rehabilitation Nurses
2506 Rose Point Road
Evanston, IL 60201
(312) 475-1000

SUMMARY

Continence clinics play a crucial role in the cure or care of individuals with incontinence. Successful clinics are established by assessing the need for the service, identifying, obtaining, and allocating resources appropriately, establishing organizational and functional activities clearly and concisely, and using comprehensive, creative promotional strategies.

Continence clinics offer opportunities for nurses to expand their role and to provide much-needed services. Nurses who are interested in establishing continence clinics or patient support groups or both should contact the identified resources for information and guidance.

SELF-EVALUATION

QUESTIONS

1. List the three phases in the process of establishing a continence clinic.
2. Identify data to be gathered in assessing the need for a continence clinic.
3. Identify resources that must be obtained before a continence clinic can be established.
4. Describe the direct and indirect services that a continence clinic provides.
5. Identify at least two target groups that should be considered in a marketing plan.
6. Identify at least four promotional strategies that can be used in marketing a continence clinic.
7. Identify the major sources of information for patients and professionals who deal with incontinence.

SELF-EVALUATION

ANSWERS

1. **a.** Development
   b. Operation
   c. Evaluation
2. **a.** Demographic data (those characteristics of the population that correlate with a high incidence of incontinence)
   b. Proximity of similar services
   c. Availability of referral sources
3. **a.** Physical plant
   b. Equipment, including diagnostic and testing equipment
   c. Personnel (physician director, nurse manager, urodynamic technician, and support personnel)
   d. Funding for the establishment of the clinic and the first 2 years of operation
   e. Referrals
4. Direct services include assessment and diagnostic workup to determine the type of incontinence, establishment of a bladder management program or treatment of incontinence, and follow-up care. Indirect services include support from social services and transportation and may include support groups.
5. **a.** Health care professionals (physicians, nurses, durable medical equipment dealers, and health maintenance organizations)
   b. Consumer groups (senior citizens' programs, retirement centers, community organizations)
6. **a.** Use of media (TV, radio, newspapers)
   b. Mail campaigns (letters to professionals, letters or questionnaires to target groups)
   c. Presentations and seminars (for professionals and for the public)
   d. Flyers
   e. Health fairs
   f. Participation in medical resource information programs
7. **a.** Simon Foundation, Inc.
   b. Help for Incontinent People (HIP)
   c. American Urological Association, Allied
   d. International Association for Enterostomal Therapy
   e. Association of Rehabilitation Nurses

REFERENCES

1. Brink C, Wells T, and Diokno A: A continence clinic for the aged, J Gerontol Nurs 9[12]:651, 1983.
2. Campbell AJ and McCosh L: Incontinence in the elderly: prevalence and prognosis, Age Aging 14:65, 1985.
3. Gross L and Bailey Z: Enterostomal therapy: developing institutional and community programs, Wakefield, Mass, 1979, Nursing Resources, Inc.
4. Herzoy A: Prevalence and incidence in a community-dwelling population. Paper presented at the NIH Consensus Conference on Urinary Incontinence in Adults, October, 1988.
5. Thomas TM et al: Prevalence of urinary incontinence, Br Med J 281:1243, 1980.

REFERENCES

6 Anatomy and Physiology of Defecation

DAVID A. ROTHENBERGER
WILLIAM J. ORROM

OBJECTIVES

1. Identify at least four factors that affect defecation and fecal continence.

2. Identify the pelvic floor muscles.

3. Explain the relationship between the external sphincter and the puborectalis muscle.

4. Differentiate the internal sphincter from the external sphincter in terms of:
   Location
   Type of musculature
   Type of innervation
   Response to rectal distention
   Role in maintaining continence

5. Define the following terms:
   Anal verge
   Dentate line
   Rectoanal inhibitory reflex
   Sampling reflex
   Rectal compliance

6. Explain the role of the intrinsic and extrinsic nervous systems in maintaining normal colon function.

7. Describe the flutter valve theory of anal sphincter function.

8. Explain the significance of the following factors in maintenance of fecal continence:
   Sensations
   Normal colonic motility
   Rectal accommodation

9. Identify three factors that affect colonic transit time.

10. Explain the role of abdominal muscle contraction (straining) in normal defecation.

The processes of fecal continence and defecation depend on a poorly understood interaction among many factors, including the psyche, diet, volume and consistency of stool, bowel motility and transit, anorectal compliance and capacity, the pelvic floor and anal sphincter function, and sensory mechanisms in the anorectum. This chapter describes the anatomic and physiologic factors critical to normal defecation and fecal continence. Changes in these aspects of anatomy and physiology can result in dysfunction and are important considerations in the treatment of fecal incontinence and defecatory disorders.

ANATOMY OF CONTINENCE AND DEFECATION
Pelvic Floor Musculature

The pelvic floor is composed of powerful sheets of muscle known as the levator ani, which stretch across the pelvis and form a diaphragm (Fig. 6-1). This diaphragm is crossed in the midline by the pelvic viscera as they exit the pelvis and descend into the perineum. The levator ani is traditionally divided into four parts: the puborectalis, the pubococcygeus, the iliococcygeus, and the ischiococcygeus. The puborectalis loops around the anorectal junction from the pubic bone and is closely associated with the external sphincter. Controversy exists as to whether the puborectalis is truly part of the levator ani complex or is more properly considered part of the external sphincter musculature. In function, at least, the puborectalis works with the deep part of the external sphincter complex.[41] The pubococcygeus also arises from the pubic bone and attaches behind the rectum to the coccyx through the postanal plate. The postanal plate, a strong musculotendinous structure composed of several layers,

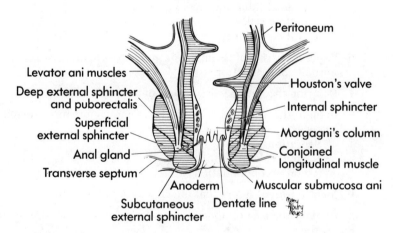

Fig. 6-1 Rectum and anal canal showing anatomic relationships among levator ani, internal sphincter, and three components of the external sphincter.

mostly fascial portions of the levator ani, lends support to the posterior portion of the anorectal region. The anterior counterpart of the postanal plate is the fibromuscular wedge of tissue known as the perineal body, which separates the posterior anal canal from the anterior urogenital viscera. The iliococcygeus arises from the ilium and the medial surface of the ischial spine. The iliococcygeus in its course overlaps the pubococcygeus and inserts below this muscle into the end of the coccyx and the anococcygeal raphe. The ischiococcygeus arises from the ischial spine and inserts into the lateral surface of the distal sacral vertebrae and proximal coccyx. The pelvic floor muscles are striated, voluntary muscles innervated through direct branches of the motor roots in the sacral vertebrae (S3-4).

Sphincter Musculature

Internal Sphincter. The internal sphincter (Fig. 6-1) is a continuation of the circular smooth muscle of the rectum. It begins at the most proximal portion of the anal canal and extends distally approximately 3 cm.[26] The internal sphincter is absent in the most distal centimeter of the anal canal. (The subcutaneous portion of the external sphincter surrounds the anal canal in this region.) Innervation to the internal sphincter is through sympathetic (excitatory) and parasympathetic (inhibitory) pathways. Since the internal sphincter is a smooth muscle, it is not under voluntary control.

External Sphincter. The external sphincter (Fig. 6-1) is a striated muscle that is divided by convention into three parts: subcutaneous, superficial, and deep. This division likely began with Santorini's description in 1715.[51] Shafik[45] proposed that the components of the external sphincter be considered three U-shaped loops (Fig. 6-2). The top (cephalad) loop consists of the deep part of the external sphincter and the puborectalis, the intermediate loop is the superficial external sphincter, and the base (caudad) loop is the subcutaneous external sphincter. From a practical standpoint, it is more convenient to divide the sphincter into superficial and deep components. The superficial muscle corresponds to the subcutaneous and superficial portions and has attachments to the coccyx through the postanal plate. The deep portion does not contact the coccyx; instead, the deep portion joins anteriorly with fibers of the puborectalis to form a functional unit, which attaches to the pubic symphysis.

Innervation of the external sphincter is through the pudendal nerve, which arises from the anterior primary rami of the second, third, and fourth sacral nerves. The external sphincter is a unique striated muscle in that it has tonic, continuous activity at rest[11]; this activity is maintained by a spinal reflex arc.[28,37,41] Another spinal reflex results in external sphincter contraction in response to rectal distention. This "initiation reflex" may be reinforced by supraspinal connections during prolonged and pronounced rectal distention.[12]

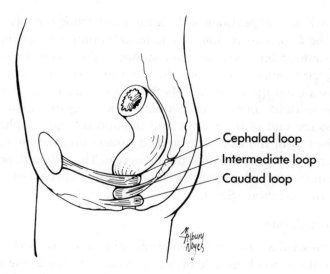

Cephalad loop
Intermediate loop
Caudad loop

Fig. 6-2 Three U-shaped components of anal sphincter mechanism as proposed by Shafik.[45]

Rectum and Anal Canal

Rectum. The rectum (Fig. 6-1) is the distal continuation of the hindgut. It differs from the sigmoid colon in its larger diameter, more complete longitudinal muscle layer, smoother mucosal lining, and three crescentic folds (Houston's valves). The rectum is 12 to 15 cm long and is divided into thirds. The upper third extends from the posterior peritoneal reflection at the rectosigmoid junction distally for 5 cm, the middle third extends from this point to the anterior reflection at about 6 to 7 cm from the distal anal canal (anal verge), and the lower third extends from the anterior reflection to the proximal anal canal. The rectum is lined with typical mucus-secreting columnar epithelium. As discussed in the following section, the type of epithelium is more variable at the junction with the anal canal.

Anal Canal. The anal canal (Fig. 6-1) is a triradiate (Y-shaped) slit with the arms of the Y lying approximately anteriorly. The distal anal canal (anal verge) is marked by the junction of the anal epithelium (anoderm) with the perianal skin. The anoderm lacks hair follicles and usually retains some pigmentation. The anal canal extends proximally to the level of the anorectal ring, where the puborectalis encircles the anorectal junction. The mucocutaneous junction is marked by the dentate line at a point 1 to 1.5 cm proximal to the anal verge; the dentate line demarcates where the endoderm of the hindgut joins the ectoderm of the skin. Distal to this line the anal canal is lined by squamous epithelium. Proximal to this line, in a transition zone that is 1 to 2 cm long, the epithelium changes from the columnar type present in the rectum to a cuboidal type, which joins the squamous epithelium of the distal anal canal.

Distal to the dentate line the anal canal is innervated by somatic nerves and is therefore sensitive to pain and touch. Above the dentate line, sensation is carried through autonomic nerves; that part of the anal canal is therefore relatively less sensitive. Above the dentate line the anal canal does have sensory nerve endings,[9] and it has been shown that the transition zone is sensitive to touch,[9] temperature changes,[29] and mild electrical stimulation.[43] Sensory stimuli in the anal transition zone may play a role in the continence mechanism,[8,29] as discussed later in this chapter.

Colon

The colon is approximately 1.2 m in length and extends from the terminal ileum to the rectum. The wall of the colon consists of an inner mucosal lining, a submucosa, and an outer layer of muscle. Peritoneum covers the colon to a variable extent throughout its course. The outer layer of muscle is composed of two layers: an inner layer, which is a continuous sheath of circular smooth muscle, and an outer longitudinal layer. The outer layer of muscle is concentrated in three narrow bands known as the teniae coli. Where the sigmoid colon approaches the rectum, these bands of muscle become more diffuse and fan out to form a continuous layer around the rectum.

The nerve supply to the colon is divided into extrinsic and intrinsic components. The extrinsic supply is through both the sympathetic and parasympathetic components of the autonomic nervous system. The parasympathetic nerve supply is through the vagus for the proximal colon and through the sacral parasympathetics for the distal colon and rectum. The sympathetic nerve supply is from the thoracolumbar outflow. The intrinsic system consists of two plexuses, one in the submucosa (the submucosal plexus, or Meissner's plexus) and one between the circular and longitudinal muscle of the colon and rectum (the myenteric plexus, or Auerbach's plexus). The extrinsic nerve supply terminates on cells in the intrinsic plexuses. If the colon is denervated by removal of the external nerve supply, it is still capable of coordinated peristalsis. Most of the smooth muscle in the colon is innervated by the intrinsic nerve supply and is modulated by the extrinsic autonomic nerves that synapse on the ganglia of the intrinsic nerves.

PHYSIOLOGY OF CONTINENCE AND DEFECATION

Normal continence and defecation depend on many factors. Maturational changes in infants result in normal continence and defecation in children. Deterioration of these complex bodily functions sometimes occurs with aging and produces significant problems in elderly individuals.

Normal Continence

Anal Sphincter Mechanism. The anal sphincter mechanism is composed of the internal and the external sphincters; these sphincters produce within the anal canal a zone of high pressure that is 3 to 5 cm long.[40] Where the anal canal joins the rectum, the puborectalis loops around behind the anorectal junction, producing an angle of approximately 60 to 105 degrees.[15] This angle is known as the anorectal angle (Fig. 6-3). The pressure within the canal at rest, when the subject is not voluntarily contracting the striated external sphincters, is mainly a result of activity of the internal sphincter. It has been shown that the internal sphincter is responsible for about 80% of resting activity.[10] The squeeze pressure in the anal canal is a result of voluntary, conscious contraction of the external sphincter and puborectalis.

There is some controversy as to how the anal sphincter mechanism contributes to continence. A theory of a "flutter" valve was described more than 20 years ago[40] and attributed continence to simple apposition of the walls of the anal canal resulting from the muscular activity of the sphincters and intra-abdominal pressure (Fig. 6-4). This theory is the most likely explanation of the anal sphincter mechanism's contribution to continence. It has also been postulated that the anorectal angle is important in maintaining continence through

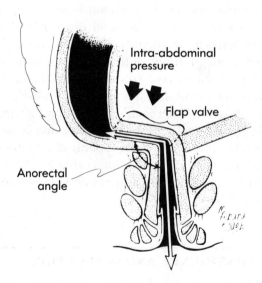

Fig. 6-3   Flap valve theory of anal continence and anorectal angle.

the mechanism of a flap valve (Fig. 6-3). It was theorized that increased intra-abdominal pressure pushes the anterior rectal wall down upon the top of the anal canal; the wall then acts as a flap that occludes the lumen and ensures continence.[13,36] However, there is little correlation between the anorectal angle and the results of operative procedures to improve continence.[20,30,31,50] During Valsalva's maneuver, the anorectal angle opens widely but the anal canal remains closed and continence is maintained, presumably because of the continuing action of the flutter valve.[3]

Sensory Factors. Distention of the rectum results in a reflex inhibition of the internal sphincter (rectoanal inhibitory reflex). The resulting drop in resting sphincter pressure allows rectal contents to come into contact with the sensitive epithelium of the proximal anal canal. This contact results in conscious recognition of rectal contents and an appropriate response to gas, liquid, or solid stool. In patients with fecal incontinence, this "sampling reflex" is impaired.[29,43] The importance of sampling is unclear: in certain operations it is completely abolished, yet continence persists.[47] The sensation of rectal fullness, which is different from the sampling reflex, is important because it alerts a person to the need to evacuate. In patients with otherwise normal sphincters, a loss of sensation secondary to neurologic injury may result in incontinence when the sphincters are overwhelmed by the unrecognized accumulation of a large volume of stool in the rectum.

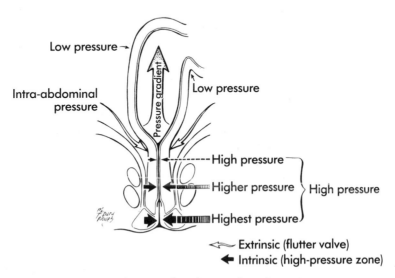

Fig. 6-4   Flutter valve theory of anal continence.

Motility Factors. The frequency of pressure waves in the anal canal has been shown to be higher in the distal anal canal than the proximal portion of the canal.[21] Such a gradient of pressure would tend to push fecal content back into the rectum and may contribute to the maintenance of complete continence. A gradient of pressure waves is also evident from the sigmoid colon to the rectum: the frequency is higher in the rectum.[6] This type of gradient would tend to impede the progress of stool into the rectum and may play a role in continence by controlling the flow of stool into the rectum.

Rectal Compliance. The "compliance" or "distensibility" of the rectum refers to the changes in pressure that occur in the rectum as the volume of stool in the rectum increases. By plotting the relationship of volume to pressure ($\Delta V/\Delta P$), the compliance can be determined. In individuals with normal rectums the maximum tolerable volume approaches 400 ml; intrarectal pressure rises to less than 20 cm H_2O.[39] In patients with poorly compliant rectums, such as in those with radiation proctitis or active inflammatory bowel disease, rapid rises in intraluminal pressure produce urgency. This urgency may lead to episodes of incontinence, especially if liquid stool, blood, and mucus are present, as they often are with these disorders.

Stool Consistency and Volume. The volume and consistency of the stool may play a more important role in continence than has been recognized previously. Normally, about 150 ml of firm feces is passed daily. When large volumes of liquid stool are rapidly emptied into the rectum, the continence mechanism may be overwhelmed; the result is incontinence. In some patients an acceptable level of continence can be restored simply by firming up the stools with a constipating agent or a bulk-increasing agent such as a psyllium seed product.

Intestinal Transit Time. Rapid transit of stool through the small intestine may result in inadequate water absorption, which may interfere with the colon's ability to dehydrate the stool to a normal consistency. The problems of liquid stool and continence have been discussed in the preceding section. Continence depends in part on the ability of the colon to store feces before they are presented to the rectum for the process of defecation. It has been shown that the sigmoid colon empties into the rectum just before defecation.[39] The sigmoid colon may therefore play a role in maintaining continence by limiting the further passage of stool until an appropriate moment for rectal evacuation arrives.

Summary. Fecal continence occurs when stool of an appropriate consistency is delivered in a regulated fashion to the rectum and sphincter musculature. Sensory awareness of rectal filling is necessary to warn of impending defecation, to determine the nature of rectal content (solid, liquid, or gas), to initiate increased contraction of the striated sphincters, and to bring about appropriate behavior. If necessary, defecation can be deferred: the rectum can accommodate the increased volume of stool. The sphincter musculature likely functions as a flutter valve with a high-pressure zone that prevents involuntary expulsion of feces and gas.

Normal Defecation

Normal defecation depends on the coordination of many factors, including the effective delivery of stool to the rectum from the colon, expulsive forces that propel the stool from the distal gastrointestinal tract, and the inhibition of the forces that maintain continence.

Intestinal Transit Time. The passage of stool obviously depends on the delivery of stool to the rectum for subsequent evacuation. Normal colonic transit has great variability; for objective assessment, it must be determined by radiologic examination. Patients are given 20 radiopaque markers at once, and radiographs of the abdomen are taken to determine the passage of these markers through the intestine. Normally, 80% of these markers are excreted in 5 days.[15] Prolonged passage of stool through the colon results in infrequent defecation and a diagnosis of constipation. This simple radiologic test using radiopaque markers confirms or refutes such a diagnosis. Transit of stool through the colon is affected by many factors, including diet, exercise, time of day, and even a person's surroundings. Eating increases the electrical and motor activity in the colon,[16] which results in a decrease in colonic transit time and increased stool frequency. Exercise has a similar effect. Increasing the bulk of the stool with fiber supplements also leads to a decrease in the intestinal transit time and can be useful in the treatment of constipation.[35]

Rectal Factors. Rectal filling normally results in cortical awareness and a call to stool. The sensory impulses resulting in cortical awareness likely arise from both the rectal wall and the surrounding musculature of the pelvic floor and sphincters. Rectal filling usually proceeds subconsciously with small rectal volumes; with the introduction of volume into the rectum the pressure in the rectum initially increases, but soon the pressure drops back to its original level. This activity is known as the accommodation response and is thought to be a result of receptive relaxation of the rectal ampulla to accommodate the fecal mass.[7] With increasing volume in the rectum an urge to defecate occurs, but the urge may disappear as accommodation occurs. As described previously, sampling of rectal contents occurs with rectal distention, and an appropriate response is initiated.

In some patients a disturbance in sensation may result in a lack of awareness of rectal filling and may contribute to constipation and eventually to fecal impaction. This distending mass of stool in the rectum results in reflex inhibition of the internal sphincter, which produces a low resting pressure and allows liquid stool to flow past the bolus of solid feces with subsequent leakage. An erroneous diagnosis of incontinence and diarrhea may result.

Whether active rectal contractions take place to expel feces is not clear. Most evidence suggests that the rectum does not actively contract but is merely an accommodating, compliant conduit for the passage of stool. Pressure waves within the rectum tend to be infrequent and of low amplitude; they do not appear to increase in frequency or amplitude as rectal filling occurs.[40] Expulsive forces likely arise from active colonic contraction, particularly in the sigmoid colon, since the sigmoid colon empties into the rectum just before rectal evacuation.[39]

Straining. Increased intra-abdominal pressure is transmitted across the surface of the bowel and imparted to the intraluminal contents of the colon and rectum. These expulsive forces are important in the process of defecation. In patients who lack the ability to contract the muscles of the abdominal wall (for example, quadriplegics), constipation is a significant problem and may be attributed in large part to the loss of this propulsive force.

Pelvic Floor and Sphincter Musculature. The point of exit of stool from the distal gastrointestinal tract is the most complicated and least understood part of the defecation process. When stool is being forced from the rectum into the anal canal, relaxation of the sphincter musculature is necessary. The internal sphincter relaxes reflexively in response to rectal distention. The external sphincter undergoes reflex contraction during the accommodation response at the time of rectal filling. When the rectum has filled sufficiently, an urge to defecate may occur; the individual may then suppress that urge or find a suitable place for defecation. When defecation takes place, a straining effort pushes the stool into the rectum, which effectively increases rectal pressure. Reflex internal sphincter relaxation occurs as expected. In this situation the external sphincter and puborectalis relax and permit passage of the stool through the anal canal. Further reflex relaxation of the external sphincter takes place as a result of stimulation of the mucosa of the anal canal by the passage of stool. Continued contraction of the puborectalis during defecation has been described; it has been proposed that this continued contraction of the puborectalis results in obstruction to fecal outflow.* This phenomenon, called the nonrelaxing puborectalis syndrome, has been implicated as a cause of constipation, but the significance of this finding is currently controversial.[18]

---

*References 1, 5, 19, 24, 42, and 48.

The role of the pelvic floor in the process of defecation is unclear. It is likely that the muscles of the pelvic floor support the anal canal and distal rectum and help transmit expulsive forces intraluminally by changing the anorectal angle. Without this support, forces applied to the enteric content through a straining effort may be dissipated by a "ballooning out" of the structures of the pelvic floor, and stool may not be evacuated effectively.

Summary. Defecation depends on the delivery of stool to the rectum through a normally functioning proximal gastrointestinal tract and colon. Expulsive forces are imposed on the intraluminal contents of the sigmoid colon and rectum by active smooth-muscle contraction in the sigmoid colon (and possibly the rectum) and by increased intra-abdominal pressure that results from a straining effort during defecation. The pelvic floor muscles support the pelvic viscera and ensure transmission of these forces beyond the pelvic floor to the intraluminal contents of the distal rectum and anal canal. As stool passes through the rectum, a coordinated relaxation of the sphincters results in a decrease in pressure in the anal canal. Rectal pressure exceeds anal canal pressure, and defecation occurs.

Maturational Changes in Continence Mechanism in Infants and Children

Anatomic and physiologic changes occur in the anorectum as infants develop. The rectum increases in length, the anal valves become apparent, and the anorectal angle becomes more acute.[14] The rectoanal inhibitory reflex is not present in premature infants. Even in infants born at full term the reflex is not present until the maturational age (gestational age plus postbirth age) exceeds 39 weeks.[17] This development coincides with the maturation of the cells of the myenteric ganglia from a bipolar to a multipolar form.[46] Until a child develops voluntary control of defecation, rectal distention results in inhibition of the external sphincter. By the age of 2½ years, maturation is associated with the development of tonic activity of the external sphincter and increased sphincter activity in response to rectal distention; this activity is mediated by a spinal reflex and augmented by supraspinal cortical centers.[32] With maturation of the sphincter, continence becomes possible.

Changes in Continence Mechanism with Age

The estimated prevalence of fecal or double (fecal and urinary) incontinence in the general population is 4.2/1000; among persons over 65 years of age the prevalence is 4.9/1000 in men and 13.3/1000 in women.[27] The problem of incontinence that occurs with aging is therefore significant. In most cases the problem of fecal incontinence is due to local factors rather than to cerebral deterioration. The most common cause is undetected fecal impaction.

The sphincter mechanism may change considerably during the course of an individual's life. These changes in the sphincter mechanism may result in dysfunction and, eventually, incontinence. The most obvious changes are those secondary to such direct trauma to the sphincters as obstetric injuries, anorectal surgery, and blunt and penetrating trauma to the perineal region. In addition, spinal cord injury may denervate the sphincters and produce incontinence that results from the loss of motor control or sensory function, or both.

The most difficult cases of fecal incontinence are those in which no obvious cause for sphincter dysfunction is evident. In these cases, which occur mainly in women, the cause is often a cumulative effect of injury during childbirth, prolonged and excessive straining during defecation, and hormonal changes. An injury that resulted in denervation has been demonstrated in the sphincter muscles of most of these patients; this type of injury probably occurs during childbirth.* Although no injury in the sphincter musculature of these patients is apparent on clinical examination, stretching of the pudendal nerve and direct sacral roots of the motor pathways may result in an injury to these structures, a "stretch neuropathy." A similar injury caused by stretching may occur during prolonged straining during defecation. A significant decline in external sphincter function has been demonstrated in women over 50 years of age when compared with younger women. No such decline is seen in men.[25] This finding is considered suggestive evidence of a hormone-dependent factor in the pelvic floor musculature in women. Changes in the hormonal milieu of the pelvic floor after menopause may result in morphologic changes in the muscle, which may in turn predispose women to incontinence, especially if underlying injury exists.

SUMMARY

Defecation and fecal continence are complex, interrelated processes that depend primarily on the interactions among the pelvic floor, the anal sphincters, the rectum, the anal canal, and the colon. The acquisition of continence depends on maturation in the innervation and anatomy of the anorectal structures. Continence depends on the orderly transit of stool of appropriate consistency and volume to the distal gastrointestinal tract, a compliant rectum that serves as an adequate storage compartment, intact sensation in the pelvic floor that alerts the individual to the need for defecation and provides information on the type of rectal content, and an adequate sphincter mechanism that can maintain anal canal pressures that are higher than pressures in the rectum. Defecation depends on the delivery of stool of an appropriate consis-

*References 2, 4, 22, 23, 33, 34, 38, 44, and 49.

tency during an appropriate period of time. Expulsive forces are necessary to propel the intraluminal contents into the rectum and, subsequently, the anal canal, while the sphincter musculature relaxes and allows content to pass. Degenerative changes occur with age and are seen mainly in women. These changes are likely the result of neurologic damage to the innervation of the sphincter musculature. Hormonal changes may also contribute to the changes seen in the pelvic floor musculature of postmenopausal women.

SELF-EVALUATION

QUESTIONS

1. Identify factors that affect defecation and fecal continence.
2. The pelvic floor musculature is collectively known as the:
   a. Puborectalis muscle
   b. Iliococcygeus muscle
   c. Levator ani muscle
   d. Perineal body
3. Explain the function of the puborectalis and its relationship to the external sphincter.
4. Nerve fibers innervating the pelvic floor come off the spinal cord at which level?
   a. T10-L2
   b. S2-4
   c. T6-8
   d. C4-6
5. Differentiate the internal sphincter from the external sphincter in terms of:
   a. Location
   b. Type of musculature
   c. Innervation
   d. Response to rectal distention
   e. Role in maintaining continence
6. Identify and discuss the significance of the following:
   a. Dentate line
   b. Anal verge
7. Describe the colon's innervation, including the role of the intrinsic and extrinsic components and their relationship.
8. Explain the flutter valve theory of anal sphincter function.
9. Identify two ways in which normal sensation contributes to fecal continence.
10. Explain the normal motility gradient between the anal canal and the sigmoid colon and its role in the maintenance of fecal continence.
11. Explain the role of rectal compliance in maintaining fecal continence.
12. Describe the effect of stool volume and consistency on fecal continence.
13. Identify the effect of the following on intestinal transit time:
    a. Eating
    b. Activity and exercise
    c. Dietary bulk
14. Explain why leakage of liquid stool may occur in patients with a fecal impaction.

15. Explain the role of abdominal muscle contraction (straining) in normal defecation.
16. Describe the physiologic changes in infants and children that make toilet training possible by about 2½ years of age.
17. Identify two factors that are thought to contribute to fecal incontinence in postmenopausal women.

SELF-EVALUATION

ANSWERS

1. Diet
   Volume and consistency of stool
   Bowel motility and transit time
   Rectal compliance and capacity
   Anorectal sensory function
   Pelvic floor and anal sphincter function
   Psyche

2. **c.** Levator ani muscle

3. The puborectalis muscle loops around the anorectal junction and attaches to the pubic symphysis; this loop creates an angle between the rectum and the anal canal. The external sphincter and puborectalis function as a unit; contraction of the external sphincter causes contraction of the puborectalis.

4. **b.** S2-4

5. **a.** The internal sphincter begins at the most proximal portion of the anal canal and extends distally for approximately 3 cm. It is absent in the most distal centimeter of the anal canal. The external sphincter surrounds the internal sphincter and also surrounds the most distal centimeter of the anal canal.

   b. The internal sphincter is a continuation of the circular smooth muscle of the rectum. The external sphincter is a striated muscle.

   c. The internal sphincter is controlled by the autonomic nervous system. (Sympathetic pathways are excitatory; parasympathetic pathways are inhibitory.) The external sphincter is controlled voluntarily; motor fibers exit the spinal cord at the sacral vertebrae (S2-4). External sphincter function is also controlled by a spinal reflex arc. The arc maintains tonic resting contraction and causes sphincter contraction in response to rectal distention.

   d. The internal sphincter relaxes in response to rectal distention; this relaxation allows the rectal contents to come into contact with the sensitive epithelium of the anal canal (sampling reflex). The external sphincter contracts in response to rectal distention (initiation reflex).

   e. The internal sphincter is primarily responsible for continence at rest; it provides 80% of resting activity. The external sphincter provides squeeze pressure, which maintains continence in the presence of rectal distention.

6. **a.** Dentate line refers to the junction between the squamous epithelium of the anal canal and the columnar epithelium of the rectum.

   b. Anal verge refers to the junction between the perianal skin and the epithelium of the anal canal (anoderm).

The lining of the anal canal distal to the dentate line (and the transition zone immediately proximal to the dentate line) is quite sensitive and provides conscious recognition of the nature of rectal contents (that is, gas, liquid, or solid). Rectal distention causes reflex relaxation of the internal sphincter, which allows rectal contents to contact the sensitive area of the proximal anal canal. This process is known as the sampling reflex.

7. The nerve supply to the colon involves both intrinsic and extrinsic components. The intrinsic system consists of Meissner's (submucosal) plexus and Auerbach's (myenteric) plexus. The extrinsic system involves fibers of the autonomic nervous system; sympathetic stimulation is inhibitory, whereas parasympathetic stimulation is excitatory.

   The extrinsic (autonomic) nerve fibers terminate on cells in the intrinsic (plexus) system. The colon is innervated primarily through the intrinsic system and is modulated by the extrinsic (autonomic) system.

   If the colon is denervated by removal of its extrinsic (autonomic) nerve supply, it remains capable of coordinated peristalsis.

8. The flutter valve theory attributes maintenance of continence to a high-pressure zone in the anal canal; this zone is created by the apposition of the walls of the anal canal that results from sphincter contraction.

9. a. Recognition of rectal fullness alerts the person to seek an appropriate time and place for defecation and to voluntarily contract the external sphincter to temporarily delay defecation.

   b. Sensory discrimination of gas, liquid, and solid permits appropriate response and management.

10. The frequency of pressure waves is higher in the anal canal than in the rectum, and the frequency of pressure waves is higher in the rectum than in the sigmoid colon. This gradient tends to slow propulsion of stool into the rectum and may support continence by controlling the flow of stool.

11. Compliance refers to the ability of the rectum to distend for low-pressure storage of stool. Normally external sphincter contraction maintains continence until the rectum adapts to accommodate the stool volume; this adaptation permits a delay in defecation. Patients with poorly compliant rectums are likely to have urgency and incontinence.

12. Normal function involves the delivery of moderate volumes of soft or solid stool to the rectum at regular intervals. Rapid delivery of large volumes of liquid stool may overwhelm the continence mechanisms. Patients with diarrhea may benefit significantly from measures to firm up the stool.

13. All three increase peristalsis, thus decreasing transit time.

14. The fecal mass produces rectal distention, which produces reflex relaxation of the internal sphincter. This relaxation allows leakage of liquid stool around the fecal bolus.

15. Abdominal muscle contraction increases intra-abdominal pressure; this pressure is transmitted to the bowel as increased intraluminal pressure, which significantly augments the propulsive forces essential for defecation.

16. Maturation of the nervous system provides tonic activity of the external sphincter and increased sphincter contraction in response to rectal distention.

17. **a.** Stretch neuropathy that results from traumatic childbirth and causes partial denervation of the pelvic floor or the sphincter mechanism or both

    b. Loss of estrogen that results in changes in pelvic floor muscles

REFERENCES

1. Barnes PRH et al: Experience of posterior division of the puborectalis muscle in the management of chronic constipation, Br J Surg 72:475, 1985.
2. Bartolo DCC et al: The role of partial denervation of the puborectalis in idiopathic fecal incontinence, Br J Surg 70:664, 1983.
3. Bartolo DCC et al: Flap-valve theory of anorectal incontinence, Br J Surg 73:1012, 1986.
4. Beersiek F, Parks AG, and Swash M: Pathogenesis of ano-rectal incontinence: a histometric study of the anal sphincter musculature, J Neurol Sci 42:111, 1979.
5. Bleijenberg G and Kuijpers HC: Treatment of the spastic pelvic floor syndrome with biofeedback, Dis Colon Rectum 30:108, 1987.
6. Connell AM: The motility of the pelvic colon. I. Motility in normals and in patients with asymptomatic duodenal ulcer, Gut 2: 175, 1961.
7. Duthie HL: Dynamics of the rectum and anus, Clin Gastroenterol 4:467, 1975.
8. Duthie HL and Bennett RC: The relation of sensation in the anal canal to the functional anal sphincter: a possible factor in anal continence, Gut 4:179, 1963.
9. Duthie HL and Gairns FW: Sensory nerve endings and sensation in the anal region of man, Br J Surg 47:585, 1960.
10. Duthie HL and Watts JM: Contribution of the external anal sphincter to the pressure zone in the anal canal, Gut 6:64, 1965.
11. Floyd WF and Walls EW: Electromyography of sphincter ani externus in man, J Physiol (Lond) 122[3]:599, 1953.
12. Frenckner B: Function of the anal sphincters in spinal man, Gut 16:638, 1975.
13. Hardcastle JD and Parks AG: A study of anal incontinence and some principles of surgical treatment, Proc R Soc Med 63:[suppl]116, 1970.
14. Hatch TF: Encopresis and constipation in children, Pediatr Clin North Am 35:257, 1988.
15. Hinton JM, Lennard-Jones JE, and Young AC: A new method for studying gut transit times using radiopaque markers, Gut 10:842, 1969.
16. Holdstock DJ et al: Propulsion (mass movements) in the human colon and its relationship to meals and somatic activity, Gut 11: 91, 1970.
17. Ito Y, Donahoe K, and Hendren WH: Maturation of the rectoanal response in premature and perinatal infants, J Pediatr Surg 12:477, 1977.
18. Jones PN et al: Is paradoxical contraction of the puborectalis of functional importance? Dis Colon Rectum 30:667, 1987.
19. Kamm MA, Hawley PR, and Lennard-Jones JE: Lateral division of the puborectalis in the management of severe constipation, Br J Surg 75:661, 1988.
20. Keighley MRB and Fielding JWL: Management of fecal incontinence and results of surgical treatment, Br J Surg 70:463, 1983.
21. Kerremans R: Morphological and physiological aspects of anal continence and defecation, Brussels, 1969, Arsica Uitgaven.

22. Kiff ES and Swash M: Normal proximal and delayed distal conduction in the pudendal nerves of patients with idiopathic (neurogenic) fecal incontinence, J Neurol Neurosurg Psychiatry 47:820, 1984.

23. Kiff ES and Swash M: Slowed conduction in the pudendal nerves in idiopathic (neurogenic) fecal incontinence, Br J Surg 71:614, 1984.

24. Kuijpers HC and Bleijenberg G: The spastic pelvic floor syndrome: a cause of constipation, Dis Colon Rectum 28:669, 1985.

25. Laurberg S and Swash M: Effects of aging on the anorectal sphincters and their innervation, Dis Colon Rectum 32:737, 1989.

26. Lawson JON and Nixon HH: Anal canal pressure in the diagnosis of Hirschsprung's disease, J Pediatr Surg 2:544, 1967.

27. Mandelstam DA: Fecal incontinence. I. Social and economic factors. In Henry MM and Swash M, eds: Coloproctology and the pelvic floor: pathophysiology and management, London, 1985, Butterworth & Co., Ltd.

28. Melzak J and Porter NH: Studies of the reflex activity of the external sphincter ani in spinal man, Paraplegia 1:277, 1964.

29. Miller R et al: Anorectal temperature sensation: a comparison of normal and incontinent patients, Br J Surg 74: 511, 1987.

30. Miller R et al: Prospective study of conservative and operative treatment for fecal incontinence, Br J Surg 75:101, 1988.

31. Miller R et al: Anterior sphincteroplasty and levatorplasty in the treatment of fecal incontinence, Br J Surg 76:1058, 1989.

32. Molander ML and Frenckner B: Electrical activity of the external anal sphincter at different ages in childhood, Gut 4:218, 1983.

33. Neill NE, Parks AG, and Swash M: Physiological studies of the anal sphincter musculature in fecal incontinence and rectal prolapse, Br J Surg 68:531, 1981.

34. Neill ME and Swash M: Increased motor unit fiber density in the external anal sphincter muscle in anorectal incontinence: a single fiber EMG study, J Neurol Neurosurg Psychiatry 43:343, 1980.

35. Painter NS, Almeida AZ, and Colebourne KW: Unprocessed bran in treatment of diverticular disease of the colon, Br Med J 11:137, 1972.

36. Parks AG, Porter NH, and Hardcastle J: The syndrome of the descending perineum, Proc R Soc Med 59: 477, 1966.

37. Parks AG, Porter NH, and Melzak J: Experimental study of the reflex mechanism controlling the muscles of the pelvic floor, Dis Colon Rectum 5:407, 1962.

38. Parks AG, Swash M, and Urich H: Sphincter denervation in anorectal incontinence and rectal prolapse, Gut 18:656, 1977.

39. Pemberton JH and Kelly KA: Achieving enteric continence: principles and applications, Mayo Clin Proc 61:586, 1986.

40. Phillips SF and Edwards AW: Some aspects of anal continence and defecation, Gut 6:396, 1965.

41. Porter NH: A physiological study of the pelvic floor in rectal prolapse, Ann Coll Surg Engl 31:379, 1962.

42. Preston DM and Lennard-Jones JE: Anismus in chronic constipation, Dig Dis Sci 30[5]:413, 1985.

43. Roe AM, Bartolo DCC, and Mortensen NJ McC: New method for assessment of anal sensation in various anorectal disorders, Br J Surg 73:310, 1986.

44. Rutter KRP: Electromyographic changes in certain pelvic floor abnormalities, Proc R Soc Med 67:53, 1974.

45. Shafik A: A concept of the anatomy of the anal sphincter mechanism and the physiology of defecation, Dis Colon Rectum 30:970, 1987.

46. Smith B: Pre and postnatal development of the ganglion cells of the rectum and its surgical implications, J Pediatr Surg 3:386, 1968.

47. Taylor BM et al: The endorectal ileal pouch–anal anastomosis: current clinical results, Dis Colon Rectum 27:347, 1984.

48. Wasserman IF: Puborectalis syndrome (rectal stenosis due to anorectal spasm), Dis Colon Rectum 7:87, 1964.
49. Womack NR, Morrison JFB, and Williams NS: The role of pelvic floor denervation in the aetiology of idiopathic fecal incontinence, Br J Surg 73:404, 1986.
50. Womack NR, Morrison JFB, and Williams NS: Prospective study of the effects of postanal repair in neurogenic incontinence, Br J Surg 75:48, 1988.
51. Wood BA: Anatomy and physiology of the anal sphincters and pelvic floor. In Henry MM and Swash M, eds: Coloproctology and the pelvic floor: pathophysiology and management, London, 1985, Butterworth & Co., Ltd.

7 Pathophysiology of Fecal Incontinence

STEPHEN B. HANAUER
KAREN S. SABLE

OBJECTIVES

1. Explain the effect of diarrheal states on fecal continence.
2. Identify at least two causes of chronic diarrhea.
3. Identify common conditions that result in neurogenic sphincter dysfunction.
4. Explain the effect of spinal cord lesions on external sphincter function.
5. Describe the effect of reduced rectal compliance on defecation patterns and continence.
6. Explain the effect of chronic rectal distention on sensation, internal sphincter function, and continence.
7. Explain why loss of normal anorectal sensation may result in fecal incontinence.
8. Describe the effect of sensory and motor neuropathies on fecal continence.
9. Identify the abnormality thought to contribute significantly to idiopathic fecal incontinence.
10. Discuss the role of behavioral components in the origin of encopresis.

Fecal incontinence is a medically benign condition; however, its social consequences can be devastating. Greater understanding of the mechanisms that maintain continence has facilitated the identification of pathophysiologic factors involved in loss of continence and has helped define specific approaches to treatment.

Anatomic and physiologic factors normally combine to maintain continence, as discussed in Chapter 6. Because many structures and processes support continence, disruption of a single mechanism may have no functional consequence.* Incontinence is frequently multifactorial, involving some compromise or impairment of multiple continence mechanisms. For example, a person with sphincter impairment may have complete continence when the stool is well formed but may have incontinence when the stool becomes liquid.

Fecal incontinence is typically neither complete nor constant, since many functional and physiologic factors affect bowel function. In addition, the degree of severity varies widely in cases of fecal incontinence; in talking with patients, it is helpful to distinguish between partial incontinence, the inability to control flatus or prevent minor soiling, and major incontinence, the inability to control stool of normal consistency.

PATHOPHYSIOLOGIC MECHANISMS

Fecal incontinence can be caused by many factors. The most common causes can be categorized as diarrhea that overwhelms the continence mechanisms, sphincter dysfunction, altered rectal compliance, anatomic alterations that affect the pelvic floor or rectum, or both, neuropathies that affect sensory function or motor function or both, skeletal and smooth muscle myopathies, and behavioral dysfunction. Causes of fecal incontinence are listed in the box on p. 191.

Diarrhea

Normal Function. Diet, motility, and secretory status determine the volume and consistency of feces presented to the rectum and the rate at which stool enters the rectum. Normally 1.0 to 1.5 liters of fluid is delivered to the colon from the ileum daily; the colon reabsorbs more than 90% of the water and converts the liquid stool to a semisolid or solid state.[21] Feces are normally retained in the sigmoid colon and propelled into the rectum intermittently; the mechanisms regulating this controlled delivery of stool to the rectum are not well understood but help to support fecal continence by preventing sudden, severe rectal distention.

Effect of Diarrhea. Stool volumes can be significantly increased as a result of increased intestinal motility, malabsorption, or secretory conditions. The individual with intact sensation, normal rectal capacity and compliance, and intact sphincter function may be able to maintain continence despite larger

---

*References 11, 13, 16, 20, 21, and 26.

CAUSES OF FECAL INCONTINENCE

ABNORMAL DELIVERY OF FECES TO RECTUM

Drug-induced (that is, cathartics, antibiotics, and so forth)
Metabolic (that is, diabetic diarrhea)
Blind loop syndrome
Inflammatory bowel disease
Infectious disease
Celiac sprue

SPHINCTER DYSFUNCTION

Trauma (disruption of nerves or musculature, surgical or obstetric trauma, or injury)
Radiation proctitis
Diabetes mellitus
Inflammatory bowel disease

REDUCED RECTAL COMPLIANCE

Rectal ischemia and fibrosis
Fecal impaction
Proctitis (inflammatory, infectious, or radiation-induced)
Infiltrating diseases or malignancy
Hirschsprung's disease

ANATOMIC DERANGEMENT

Obstetric or surgical trauma
Injury
Congenital malformations of anorectum
Inflammatory bowel disease (that is, fistula, abscess, or perianal disease)
Rectal prolapse
Third-degree hemorrhoids
Tumor

NEUROLOGIC IMPAIRMENT

Central nervous system
   Stroke
   Trauma
   Tumor
   Degenerative disease (that is, dementia)
   Encephalopathy
   Mental retardation
   Psychiatric disorders (that is, depressive disorders)
   Drug reaction or intoxication
Spinal
   Multiple sclerosis
   Tumor
   Trauma
   Meningomyelocele (spina bifida)
   Degenerative disease (that is, severe vitamin B_{12} deficiency)
Peripheral nervous system
   Diabetes (polyneuropathy)
   Shy-Drager syndrome
   Tabes dorsalis
   Cauda equina lesions
   Guillain-Barré syndrome
   Toxic neuropathy
   Idiopathic fecal incontinence
   Perineal descent syndrome

MUSCULAR AND NEUROMUSCULAR DISORDERS

Congenital or hereditary myopathy
Myasthenia gravis
Idiopathic fecal incontinence
Perineal descent syndrome

BEHAVIORAL AND DEVELOPMENTAL DYSFUNCTIONS

Childhood encopresis?
Mental retardation
Psychiatric disorders (rarely)

stool volumes and precipitous delivery of stool to the rectum. In other individuals diarrhea may overwhelm the continence mechanisms. In such cases the investigation and management of fecal incontinence should be directed toward controlling or treating the underlying causes of diarrhea.

Causative Factors. There are many possible causes of diarrhea. A careful history may reveal the use of medications that can exacerbate or cause diarrhea (for example, antacids, cathartics, prokinetic agents, or antibiotics) or the excessive consumption of nonabsorbed carbohydrates (for example, sorbitol).

Diseases of the small bowel must be considered in evaluating and managing diarrhea. Diabetes is one disease that can result in diarrhea: 10% to 20% of patients with long-standing diabetes have diarrhea associated with autonomic neuropathy. One hypothesis is that motility disorders cause reduced transit time, which limits the absorption of bile salts in the small bowel; the diarrhea that results is secondary to rapid transit and to the irritant effect of bile acids on the colon (choleretic diarrhea).[19a] An alternative theory is that altered motility may cause stasis: bacterial overgrowth then causes the diarrhea.[19a] Other studies have indicated that diabetic diarrhea may be caused by disruption of alpha$_2$-adrenergic receptors that normally promote fluid and electrolyte absorption and inhibit anion secretion. The implications for treatment are (1) that glucose levels must be rigidly controlled to minimize the neuropathy thought to contribute to motility disorders and (2) that the use of alpha$_2$-adrenergic agonists (for example, clonidine or lidamidine) can reduce the volume and frequency of stools and may also slow gastrointestinal transit.[4,7,19,22] Other factors that may contribute to diarrhea in the patient with diabetes include altered colonic motility, abnormal rectal sensation, and altered anal sphincter function.

Other causes of diarrhea include inflammatory bowel disease, infectious disease, radiation enteritis, and malabsorption syndromes. For any patient with diarrhea the initial goal is to determine the cause; therapy is then directed toward eliminating causative factors and implementing measures to reduce fecal volume, improve stool consistency, and reduce frequency of defecation and incontinence.

Sphincter Dysfunction

Internal Sphincter. Anal sphincter tone depends on both internal and external sphincter mechanisms. The internal anal sphincter is responsible for the majority of the anal canal's resting pressure.[10,21] This tonic, involuntary contraction is related to the intrinsic innervation of the smooth muscle and the interplay of autonomic nerves. As discussed in Chapter 6, rectal distention normally causes reflex relaxation of the internal sphincter. This reflex, mediated by the intrinsic neural plexus of the rectum, is absent in Hirschsprung's disease; in these patients large masses of stool typically accumulate above the aganglionic bowel and closed internal sphinter, and liquid stool may leak around the fecal bolus.

The importance of the internal anal sphincter in maintaining continence is controversial. Schiller thinks that damage to the internal sphincter (or even transection) results in only a modest compromise of fecal continence.[21] Other authors attach more importance to the role of the internal sphincter in maintaining continence.[10] The internal sphincter may be compromised by several diseases or traumatic conditions, including radiation proctitis, diabetes mellitus, perianal Crohn's disease, and anal dilatation for treatment of hemorrhoids. Loss of internal sphincter function alone may induce partial incontinence; the patient who also has diarrhea may have major incontinence.

External Sphincter. The external anal sphincter provides voluntary control by means of both tonic and phasic activity; this activity is mediated by the pudendal nerve (sacral cord S3-4), which innervates the striated sphincter muscle. Distention of the rectum with feces stimulates contraction of the external anal sphincter, which increases pressure in the lower anal canal. External sphincter contraction also results in contraction of the puborectalis muscle, which pulls forward and produces a right angle between the rectum and the anal canal, further impeding the movement of feces.[10,14] The phasic increase in the external sphincter activity lasts only seconds, whereas voluntary efforts can be maintained for about 1 minute. Thus the external anal sphincter is able to delay defecation for only a short time; continence beyond this point depends on the rectum's ability to accommodate the increased volume (rectal compliance).

Dysfunction of the external sphincter alone usually causes a minor degree of incontinence. When both the external sphincter and the puborectalis muscles are compromised, more severe incontinence develops. Such dysfunction is most often due to traumatic injury or neurologic impairment. Injury caused by impalement, pelvic fracture, or obstetric or surgical damage may result in disruption of the sphincter musculature and/or damage to the pudendal or sacral nerve branches, which innervate the external sphincter and puborectalis muscles.[23]

Neurologic compromise originating in the central nervous system may impair sensory function or voluntary sphincter control or both. Cerebrovascular disease, tumors, degenerative disorders, or drug intoxication are common causes of neurologic compromise; altered sensorium as a result of medication is a common cause of loss of sphincter control in elderly individuals.

Spinal cord lesions (for example, multiple sclerosis, tumors, or injuries) reduce the patient's ability to contract the external sphincter in response to rectal distention (when the internal sphincter reflexively relaxes and continence depends on external sphincter contraction). In these patients continence usually depends on the maintenance of formed stool and a regular bowel evacuation program: such patients are unable to control liquid stool or unexpected stools.

Altered Rectal Compliance

When feces enter and distend the rectum, intrarectal pressures rise and the urge to defecate is felt. Normal compliance and relaxation of the rectal vault result in a reduction of the intraluminal pressure and thus reduce the urge to defecate. An intact enteric nervous system and functioning smooth muscle are necessary for rectal compliance so that the rectum functions as a reservoir.

Reduced Compliance. In patients with reduced rectal compliance, a given volume of fecal material results in higher intrarectal pressures at an earlier stage of rectal filling. Storage time is shortened, rectal urgency is common, and fecal incontinence may result, if the patient is unable to reach a toilet quickly. (As discussed earlier in this chapter, the external sphincter can be contracted maximally only for about 1 minute; continence beyond this point depends on rectal compliance, which correlates with a decrease in rectal pressure.)

In some elderly patients, rectal pressures are high because of loss of tissue elasticity associated with rectal ischemia and fibrosis.[6] Reduced rectal compliance is also present in cases of infectious proctitis, infiltrating or obstructing malignancies, chronic rectal ischemia, radiation proctitis, and inflammatory bowel disease.[11,20,21,26]

Hirschsprung's disease, or congenital aganglionosis of the distal colon, may also lead to loss of rectal compliance. Failure of caudal migration (or subsequent axonic damage) of ganglion cells results in a denervated segment that remains in a state of tonic, uninhibited contraction[3]; also, the internal sphincter fails to relax in response to rectal distention, as discussed earlier in this chapter. Failure of rectal and internal sphincter relaxation may produce functional obstruction with leakage of liquid stool around an impacted fecal mass. Although Hirschsprung's disease typically involves the rectosigmoid, shorter or longer bowel segments can also be involved. Clinical presentation depends on the extent of involvement and may vary from the commonly seen condition of obstipation to fecal incontinence.[3,21]

Increased Compliance. Conversely, chronic distention of the rectum from impacted stool can result in excessive rectal compliance (stretch) and persistent stimulation of the rectoanal inhibitory reflex. This chronic distention can eventually result in impaired sensation and sphincter dysfunction, with loss of the ability to retain liquid stool.[17] In addition, bacterial action leads to liquefaction of feces proximal to the impaction. Liquid stool then leaks around the impaction through lax sphincters and results in fecal soiling.[25] A rectal examination is necessary to differentiate between impaction and continued soiling from diarrhea; in the patient with impaction, digital examination usually reveals a lax anal sphincter and a rectum full of formed feces.

Anatomic Alterations

Anatomic disruption of the pelvis or rectum is a common cause of fecal incontinence and most often results from obstetric trauma or surgical procedures. Congenital malformations of the anus and rectum are rare causes of anatomic sphincter deficiency.

Anatomic abnormalities may result from destruction or injury of the internal or external sphincter, loss of the normal anorectal angle, or impairment of rectal capacity, compliance, or contractility. Again, loss of a single mechanism may not induce fecal incontinence unless the loss is compounded by diarrhea or disruption of a second mechanism.

Neuropathies

Sensory Neuropathy. Anorectal sensation allows most individuals to differentiate between gas, liquid, and solid matter in the rectum. The mechanism by which this discrimination reaches a conscious level is not understood. Rectal sensation is regulated by autonomic and somatic responses to rectal distention, and several different receptors and pathways may be involved. Autonomic responses are organized through the myenteric plexus and may also involve reflex arcs to the spinal cord. The perception of rectal distention may also be mediated by stretch receptors in muscles of the pelvic diaphragm; such perception requires intact somatic nerve pathways and an intact central nervous system.[*] The individual with normal sensation perceives rectal distention and can then contract the external sphincter and pelvic floor muscles to delay defecation. Impaired anorectal sensation removes the signal that warns of impending defecation and may result in incontinence.

Defective pelvic or anorectal sensation may result from a variety of central or peripheral neuropathies. Patients with altered mentation caused by stroke, encephalopathy, or dementia often are unable to recognize or respond to normal rectal stimuli. Similarly, patients with depressive psychiatric disorders, mental retardation, brain tumors, or tabes dorsalis may fail to respond to appropriate stimuli. Rectal sensation may also be impaired in patients with other neurologic conditions such as multiple sclerosis, meningomyelocele (spina bifida), and Shy-Drager syndrome.

Metabolic derangements can also affect anorectal sensation. More than 50% of patients with fecal incontinence caused by diabetes have impaired rectal sensation without loss of rectal compliance or a change in the threshold for

---

*References 1, 11, 13, 16, 20, 21, and 26.

internal sphincter relaxation.[26] In contrast, sensation is normal in patients with diabetes who do not have fecal incontinence, which suggests that intact rectal sensation may be an important factor in maintaining continence.

Mixed Sensorimotor Neuropathies. Multiple sclerosis and spinal cord injury are examples of neurologic disorders that can impair both sensory and motor function. Multiple sclerosis is a common neurologic disease characterized by focal demyelination of axons within any area of the white matter of the brain or spinal cord. In a recent survey, 51% of patients with multiple sclerosis reported fecal incontinence; fecal incontinence was common even in mild cases, increased with decreasing mobility, and correlated strongly with the presence of genitourinary symptoms.[15] Both sensory and motor pathways are affected, leading to multifactorial fecal incontinence. Abnormal colonic motility and loss of the gastrocolic reflex have been demonstrated in patients with multiple sclerosis; these conditions affect peristalsis and stool consistency. These patients also have impaired anorectal sensation and denervation of the external anal sphincter; perception of rectal distention is therefore less acute in these patients, and the ability to delay defecation by contracting the external sphincter is reduced.[15]

In patients with spinal cord injury or meningomyelocele, the severity of the impairment is determined by the level of the defect and the degree of neural involvement. Frequently these patients have alterations in sensory perception and in external sphincter control, caused by interrupted neural pathways. These patients may be unable to sense or respond to rectal distention; therefore continence usually depends on maintenance of formed stools and a regular program for bowel evacuation.

Motor Neuropathy. Neuropathies may also lead to a motor deficit. For example, despite normal sensory innervation, spinal cord lesions at the sacral level (S2-4) result in a motor deficit that affects urinary and fecal continence: the motor nerves are interrupted, although sensory nerves remain intact. Other syndromes may result in fecal incontinence, including Guillain-Barré postinfectious syndrome, which results in motor dysfunction and possibly autonomic dysfunction, and vitamin B_{12} deficiency, which causes subacute combined degeneration of the spinal cord. Myasthenia gravis and a wide variety of other rare neurologic syndromes may also predispose the patient to fecal incontinence caused by impaired nerve function. In addition, most patients with "idiopathic" fecal incontinence have been found to have neuropathic changes of the external sphincter and pelvic floor musculature.[2,18]

Skeletal and Smooth-Muscle Myopathies

Colonic motility, sphincter tone, and the anorectal angle[13,20,21,26] are normally maintained by basal muscle tone; the exact mechanism is not known but is thought to be part of the spinal reflex. In addition, rectal and pelvic sensation contribute to the control of fecal evacuation by triggering neural stimuli that result in the contraction or relaxation of skeletal and smooth muscle.

Abnormal skeletal muscle function is thought to be a major cause of idiopathic fecal incontinence. Histopathologic and electromyographic studies reveal denervation of the puborectalis and external anal sphincter muscles[26]; such denervation occurs in the perineal descent syndrome, in which repeated stretching of the perineal musculature injures both the muscles and the associated motor nerves. Progressive denervation leads to further weakness of the pelvic diaphragm, although continence usually is not impaired unless both the external sphincter and puborectalis are damaged.[11,26]

Similarly, neuromuscular damage may occur in women during childbirth. Prolonged labor may damage motor nerves to the muscles of the pelvic diaphragm and the anal sphincters. In addition, perineal tears may actually disrupt the sphincter muscles themselves. Multiparous women are more prone to these problems because injury may be repeated; such damage is frequently associated with rectal prolapse.

Congenital and hereditary myopathies are rare causes of fecal incontinence. Often it is not clear whether an actual muscular abnormality exists or whether the patient's lack of mobility (inability to reach the toilet) results in incontinence. In such cases anal manometry may be helpful in determining the cause of the incontinence.

Behavioral Dysfunction

The role of behavioral problems in fecal incontinence and the psychogenic and psychiatric components that contribute to fecal incontinence have been studied extensively in children with encopresis and constipation. Fecal incontinence in children is usually related to constipation and recurrent fecal impaction. Some researchers have theorized that active withholding occurs[12]; however, physiologic causes must be ruled out. Some studies have identified an increased incidence of developmental delay and deficits in mentation in children with constipation and fecal incontinence[12] and a higher incidence of learning disabilities in children with encopresis.[24] In contrast, Friman found that children with constipation and fecal incontinence did not have a significantly higher incidence of behavioral problems.[9] Although many children with encopresis are found to have no demonstrable learning or behavioral problems, constipation and encopresis are common in children with moderate to severe mental retardation.

Although learning disabilities and cognitive disabilities have been identified in some children with encopresis and constipation, no clear-cut association with psychiatric disorders has been found in children or adults with fecal incontinence.[8] On the other hand, there are case reports of fecal incontinence in patients with obsessive-compulsive disorders or severe depression. Treatment of the underlying psychiatric disorders in these patients along with attention to the possible constipating effects of some antidepressants can lead to resolution of incontinence.

SUMMARY

An intricate and complex interaction among anatomic, neurologic, and muscular processes maintains normal fecal continence. Depending on the quality and quantity of stool, interruption of a single mechanism or multiple mechanisms can induce fecal soilage. Sphincter function, rectal compliance, maintenance of anatomic structure, neuromuscular function, and normal volition are essential. Disruptive pathophysiology often affects multiple processes.

Understanding the underlying pathophysiology that results in fecal incontinence has important therapeutic implications. As discussed in the following chapters, treatment strategies that may be beneficial in some cases are of little use in others. Understanding of altered continence mechanisms provides the basis for prevention or correction of fecal incontinence.

SELF-EVALUATION

QUESTIONS

1. Identify at least four causes of fecal incontinence.
2. Explain the effect of diarrhea on fecal continence.
3. Identify at least three possible causes of diarrhea.
4. Explain the effect of Hirschsprung's disease on internal sphincter function.
5. Explain the effect of spinal cord lesions on external sphincter function and fecal continence.
6. Explain the importance of compliance in maintaining fecal continence.
7. Anatomic alteration in pelvic floor structures is most commonly due to:
    a. Congenital anomalies
    b. Impalement injuries
    c. Obstetric injuries
    d. Normal deterioration associated with aging
8. Explain the significance of impaired anorectal sensation as a causative factor in fecal incontinence.
9. Explain the effect of neurologic dysfunction on continence mechanisms, including sensory function and motor function.
10. Common causes of neurogenic incontinence include:
    a. Multiple sclerosis and spinal cord lesions
    b. Congenital and hereditary myopathies
    c. Operative trauma
    d. Psychiatric and behavioral disorders
11. Idiopathic incontinence is commonly related to:
    a. Psychogenic factors
    b. Cognitive disorders
    c. Damage to pelvic floor musculature
    d. Motility disorders
12. Behavioral dysfunction has been shown to be the primary etiologic factor for encopresis.
    a. True
    b. False

SELF-EVALUATION

ANSWERS

1. **a.** Diarrhea that overwhelms continence mechanisms
   b. Sphincter dysfunction
   c. Compromised rectal compliance
   d. Anatomic abnormalities of the pelvis or rectum
   e. Altered anorectal sensation
   f. Myopathies that affect the pelvic floor muscles
   g. Behavioral dysfunction

2. Diarrhea results in large volumes of liquid stool being delivered precipitously to the rectum. The patient with normal continence mechanisms detects rectal distention and is able to contract the external sphincter to delay defecation. Maximal contraction of the external sphincter can be maintained for about 1 minute; continence beyond this point depends on the rectum's ability to adapt. With large volumes of liquid stool, the rectum's ability to adapt may be overwhelmed; in this case, continence depends on the proximity of toilet facilities.

   The patient with any compromise of continence mechanisms (sensory awareness, sphincter function, or rectal compliance) is likely to become incontinent during episodes of diarrhea.

3. **a.** Medications
   b. Malabsorption syndromes
   c. Inflammatory conditions of the bowel
   d. Infectious diseases of the bowel
   e. Diabetes

4. Normally the internal sphincter relaxes in response to rectal distention. In Hirschsprung's disease, loss of normal innervation results in loss of this reflex; the internal sphincter remains contracted in the presence of rectal distention and contributes to a functional obstruction.

5. The patient is unable to contract the external sphincter voluntarily in response to rectal distention. Continence in these patients usually depends on the maintenance of formed stool (a passively contracted sphincter is competent for formed stool but not for liquid stool) and a regular bowel elimination program. These patients are unable to control liquid stool or unexpected stool.

6. Normal compliance means the rectum is able to stretch and store stool at low pressures.

   When a bolus of stool enters the rectum, the intrarectal pressure rises and threatens continence. Normally the individual senses rectal distention and contracts the external sphincter and puborectalis, thereby increasing the anal canal pressure and maintaining continence. The external sphincter can be contracted maximally for only about 1 minute; relaxation of the sphincter then occurs and reduces anal canal pressure. Continence beyond this point depends on the rectum's ability to stretch and accommodate the stool. With normal compliance the rectum stretches and the intrarectal pressure drops so that continence is maintained.

The patient with poor compliance has the sensation of extreme urgency and may be incontinent.

7. **c.** Obstetric injuries

8. Recognition of rectal distention allows the individual to contract the external sphincter and pelvic floor so that continence is maintained. Loss of this protective mechanism predisposes the individual to incontinence.

9. Neurologic lesions can impair sensory function or motor function or both. The severity of impairment ranges from mild dysfunction to total loss of function.

Sensory dysfunction causes partial or total loss of the ability to detect rectal distention and recognize impending defecation.

Motor dysfunction causes partial or total loss of the ability to control the external sphincter and delay or initiate defecation.

10. **a.** Multiple sclerosis and spinal cord injuries

11. **c.** Damage to pelvic floor musculature

12. **b.** False

REFERENCES

1. Allen ML, Orr WC, and Robinson MG: Anorectal functioning in fecal incontinence, Dig Dis Sci 33:36, 1988.
2. Bartolo DCC et al: The role of partial denervation of the puborectalis in idiopathic fecal incontinence, Br J Surg 70:664, 1983.
3. Blisard KS and Kleinman R: Hirschsprung's disease: a clinical and pathologic overview, Hum Pathol 17:1189, 1986.
4. Chang EB, Fedorak R, and Field M: Experimental diabetic diarrhea in rats: intestinal mucosal denervation hypersensitivity and treatment with clonidine, Gastroenterology 91:564, 1986.
5. Denis P et al: Elastic properties of the rectal wall in normal adults and in patients with ulcerative colitis, Gastroenterology 77:45, 1979.
6. Devroede G et al: Ischemic fecal incontinence and rectal angina, Gastroenterology 83:970, 1982.
7. Fedorak RN, Field M, and Chang EB: Treatment of diabetic diarrhea with clonidine, Ann Intern Med 102:197, 1985.
8. Fisher SE et al: Psychiatric screening for patients with fecal incontinence or chronic constipation referred for surgical treatment, Br J Surg 76:352, 1989.
9. Friman PC et al: Do encopretic children have clinically significant behavior problems? Pediatrics 82:407, 1988.
10. Gonella J, Bouvier M, and Blanquet F: Extrinsic nervous control of motility of small and large intestines and related sphincters, Physiol Rev 67:902, 1987.
11. Hanauer SB: Fecal incontinence in the elderly, Hosp Pract, p 105, March 1988.
12. Hatch TF: Encopresis and constipation in children, Pediatr Clin North Am 35:257, 1988.
13. Henry MM: Pathogenesis and management of fecal incontinence in the adult, Gastroenterol Clin North Am 16:35, 1987.
14. Henry MM and Thomson JPS: The anal sphincter, Scand J Gastroenterol 93[Suppl]:53, 1984.
15. Hinds JP and Wald A: Colonic and anorectal dysfunction associated with multiple sclerosis, Am J Gastroenterol 84:587, 1989.
16. Pemberton JH and Kelly KA: Achieving enteric continence: principles and applications, Mayo Clin Proc 61:586, 1986.
17. Read NW and Abouzekry L: Why do patients with fecal impaction have fecal incontinence? Gut 27:283, 1986.
18. Rogers J et al: Pelvic floor neuropathy: a comparative study of diabetes mellitus and idiopathic fecal incontinence, Gut 29:756, 1988.
19. Roof LW: Treatment of diabetic diarrhea with clonidine, Am J Med 83:603, 1987.
19a. Sable KS and Chang EM: Treating GI complications in the diabetic patient, Drug Ther, p 63, Aug 1989.
20. Schiller LR: Fecal incontinence, Clin Gastroenterol 15:687, 1986.
21. Schiller LR: Fecal incontinence. In Sleissenger MH and Fordtran JS, eds: Gastrointestinal disease, ed 4, Philadelphia, 1989, WB Saunders Co.
22. Schiller LR et al: Studies of the antidiarrheal action of clonidine: effects of motility and intestinal absorption, Gastroenterology 89:982, 1985.
23. Snooks SJ, Henry MM, and Swash M: Fecal incontinence due to external anal sphincter division in childbirth is associated with damage to the innervation of the pelvic floor musculature: a double pathology, Br J Obstet Gynaecol 92:824, 1985.
24. Stern HP et al: The incidence of cognitive dsyfunction in an encopretic population in children, Neurotoxicology 9[3]:351, 1988.
25. Tobin GW: Incontinence in the elderly, Practitioner 231:843, 1987.
26. Wald A: Disorders of defecation and fecal continence, Cleve Clin J Med 56:491, 1989.

8 Assessment of Patients with Fecal Incontinence

JAMES H. MacLEOD

OBJECTIVES

1. Describe the normal sequence of events that maintains continence in the presence of rectal distention.
2. Identify the motor structures that must be assessed in the patient with fecal incontinence.
3. Identify at least two objectives in the assessment of a patient with fecal incontinence.
4. Describe the data concerning bowel function and fecal incontinence that are gathered during the initial patient interview.
5. Explain the relationship between diarrhea and fecal incontinence and the implications for the assessment of patients with diarrhea.
6. List three body systems that are included in a focused review of systems and surgical history for the patient with fecal incontinence.
7. Identify commonly used prescription drugs and over-the-counter drugs that may affect fecal continence by altering bowel motility or stool consistency.
8. Identify information to be included in a bowel function diary.
9. Describe data to be obtained from a visual and digital examination of the anus and rectum.
10. Describe the procedure for each of the following studies and data to be gained from each:
    Defecography
    Balloon sphincterography
    Ultrasonography

11. Identify the three components of continence that can be assessed with anorectal manometry.

12. Describe the normal sensory threshold for rectal distention in terms of volume and time.

13. Describe a normal anorectal study in terms of internal sphincter response to rectal distention and external sphincter response to rectal distention.

14. Identify data to be gained from sphincter electromyography.

15. Identify normal rectal capacity as measured by the balloon reservoir study.

16. Explain the relevance of the patient's (or caregiver's) goals, motivation, and support systems to the assessment and management of fecal incontinence.

Thorough assessment of the patient with fecal incontinence is necessary to identify the causative and contributing factors, which in turn direct the treatment plan. Accurate assessment depends on an understanding of the normal continence mechanisms and the diseases or conditions that can disrupt these mechanisms.

NORMAL FUNCTION AS BASIS FOR ASSESSMENT

The mechanism of fecal continence is complex and consists of several coordinated components. Since our understanding of this mechanism has improved in recent years, it is now possible, albeit still difficult, to evaluate each of these components separately and to appropriately treat the one that is deficient.

Anatomic Structures

Motor Structures. Continence is normally maintained by an interplay between smooth-muscle structures and striated muscle structures. The internal sphincter is a smooth-muscle structure that surrounds the anal canal; it is a condensation of the distal fibers of the involuntary, circular muscle of the rectum.

The voluntary (striated) anal musculature is a continuous sheet of muscle that extends from the floor of the pelvis to the anal verge; the anal musculature consists of the levator ani, puborectalis, and external anal sphincter (Fig. 8-1). The puborectalis blends with the levator ani, which is above it, and the external sphincter, which is below it. Its fibers pass posteriorly from the pubic symphysis to both sides of the anorectum. The fibers meet behind the anorectum (Fig. 8-2) to form a sling. This sling pulls the alimentary canal anteriorly so that the

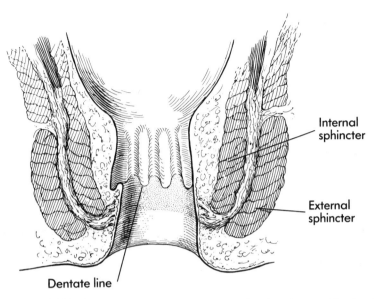

Fig. 8-1   Section of anorectum showing musculature. (From MacLeod JH: A method of proctology, New York, 1979, Harper & Row, Publishers, Inc, p 4.)

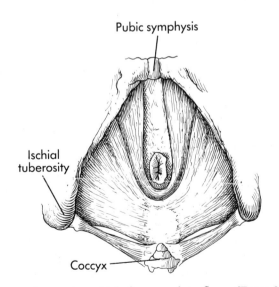

Fig. 8-2   Levator ani muscle, which forms pelvic floor. (From MacLeod JH: A method of proctology, New York, 1979, Harper & Row, Publishers, Inc, p 4.)

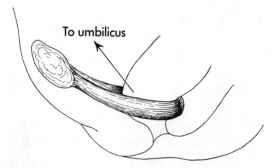

To umbilicus

Fig. 8-3 Sagittal section showing puborectalis sling. (From MacLeod JH: A method of proctology, New York, 1979, Harper & Row, Publishers, Inc, p 5.)

axis of the anal canal lies at a right angle to that of the rectum (Fig. 8-3), thus forming the important anorectal angle. The puborectalis is deficient anteriorly; therefore a laceration in this area is likely to cause incontinence, especially in a parous woman.

The external sphincter forms a ring that surrounds the distal 2 cm of the anal canal; the superficial portion of the external sphincter is attached posteriorly to the coccyx and anteriorly to the perineal body. The external sphincter lies outside the internal sphincter.

Sensory Structures. The dentate line (Fig. 8-1), an important landmark, lies at the midpoint of the anal canal; it forms the junction between mucosa and skin and roughly delineates the boundary between autonomic and somatic nerve supply. Innervation above the dentate line is autonomic, and sensation above the line is limited to that caused by stretching; the area below the dentate line is somatically innervated and contains an abundant supply of nerve endings that are exquisitely sensitive to touch, pain, and temperature. Sensory discrimination of gas, liquid, and solid takes place in this area below the dentate line.[5]

Physiology of Continence

Continence at Rest. Continence at rest is maintained by tonic contraction of all the sphincter muscles; the internal sphincter is maximally contracted at rest, and the external sphincter and puborectalis are minimally contracted (even during sleep).[3,4] Internal sphincter contraction at rest prevents the leakage of volumes of fluid or flatus so small (1 ml or less) as to be otherwise undetectable. In most people, the role of the internal sphincter can be assumed by the voluntary muscles (for example, after internal sphincterotomy).[15,20] The external sphincter and puborectalis contract further in response to perianal stimulation, postural changes, increases in intra-abdominal pressure, and rectal distention.[3]

Table 8-1 Physiology of fecal continence

Component	Innervation	Role
SENSORY		
Rectal sensation	Autonomic	Warning of rectal filling
Anal sensation	Somatic	Sampling of rectal contents; discrimination of gas, liquid, and solid; warning of breach of continence mechanism
MOTOR		
External sphincter (and perineal body)	Somatic	Lateral closure
Puborectalis (anorectal angle)	Somatic	Lateral closure
Internal sphincter	Autonomic	Relaxation with rectal distention; contraction at rest; fine-tuning of continence
RESERVOIR		
Rectal capacity and compliance	Autonomic	Retention of adequate volume; distensibility without increase in pressure
Colon motility	Autonomic	Maintenance of volume and consistency of stool

From MacLeod JH: Endoscopy Rev 5:45, 1988.

Response to Rectal Distention. The mechanisms of continence are listed in Table 8-1 and diagrammed in Fig. 8-4. These mechanisms are fully set into action by rectal distention, which results in the following:

1. A sense of fullness, which is mediated by autonomic nerve endings outside the rectum in the levator ani.[4,9] This sense of fullness acts as a signal to the individual to contract the external sphincter. Impairment of this sensation removes the warning signal that defecation is imminent.

2. Internal sphincter relaxation, which allows anal sampling to occur.[14,20] Rectal contents come into contact momentarily with the lining of the upper anal canal, where discrimination among gas, liquid, and solid takes place and warning is given of any impending breach of the continence mechanism. So abundant is the innervation of the upper anal canal that flatus can be identified and selectively passed.

3. Voluntary contraction of the external sphincter and puborectalis in response to both rectal distention and anal sampling. These muscles close the anal canal by lateral compression and render the anorectal angle more acute (Fig. 8-5).[15,20] These muscles must be innervated, must be at

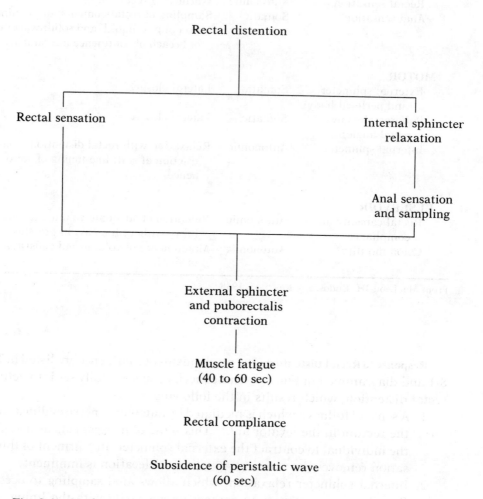

Fig. 8-4 Mechanisms of fecal continence. (From MacLeod JH: Endoscopy Rev 5:45, 1988.)

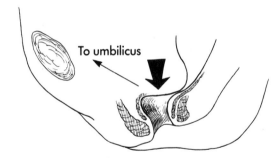

Fig. 8-5   Acute angulation between anal canal and rectum and anorectal flap valve. (From MacLeod JH: A method of proctology, New York, 1979, Harper & Row, Publishers, Inc, p 86.)

least partially intact, and must contract as one against an intact perineum.

4. However, the external sphincter and puborectalis can contract maximally for only 40 to 60 seconds[4]; continence beyond that point depends on the reservoir function of the rectum, which includes both an adequate capacity (300 to 500 ml) and adequate compliance (that is, the rectum's ability to distend to accommodate oncoming stool without a corresponding increase in intrarectal pressure until the peristaltic wave subsides, which, fortunately, occurs in less than 60 seconds).[4]

Stool volume and consistency and bowel transit time are secondary factors in the maintenance of continence and must also be assessed.

PATHOPHYSIOLOGY OF INCONTINENCE

The causes of fecal incontinence are discussed in Chapter 7 and categorized in the box on p. 191. Their pathophysiologic effects are shown in Table 8-2.

As stated in previous chapters, the condition of continence is relative, not "all or none." The most competent sphincter apparatus is not necessarily proof against a sudden, explosive diarrhea. Conversely, when the sphincter complex is grossly deficient or a large portion of the rectum has been removed, continence may still be maintained if the bowel functions to deliver firm feces only once or twice daily. However, if the patient with a deficient sphincter also has an irritable bowel or if the patient who has already had a rectal resection has further anorectal surgery, continence is less likely. Thus assessment and management of the patient with fecal incontinence must include attention to every factor that affects bowel function and fecal continence.

Table 8-2   Pathophysiologic effects of fecal incontinence

Component	Cause
SENSORY	
Rectal sensation	Degenerative
	Diabetes
	Neurogenic disease or disorder
	Impaction
Anal sensation	Traumatic (scarring)
	Diminished discrimination and control of flatus, and seepage
MOTOR	
External sphincter and puborectalis	Congenital
	Traumatic
	Operative injury
	Obstetric injury
	Penetrating wound
	Inflammatory
	Neoplastic
	Degenerative
	Prolapse
	Neurogenic
	Idiopathic
Internal sphincter	Traumatic
	Operative injury
RESERVOIR	
Rectal capacity and compliance	Traumatic
	Surgery (anterior resection, coloanal anastomosis, especially if septic)
	Radiation
	Ischemia
	Inflammatory bowel disease
Colon capacity and motility	Colon disease or resection

From MacLeod JH: Endoscopy Rev 5:45, 1988.

ASSESSMENT OF PATIENTS WITH FECAL INCONTINENCE
Objectives of Assessment

In assessing the patient with fecal incontinence, the practitioner must remain aware that the ultimate objective is to establish an effective treatment plan for elimination or management of the incontinence. During assessment, therefore, the practitioner must identify the factors that are contributing to the incontinence and the factors that may affect treatment. Specifically, the objective of assessment is to identify the following:

1. Cause or causes of the incontinence
2. Component of the continence mechanism that is affected (that is, sensory, motor, or reservoir)
3. Degree (or severity) of the incontinence
4. Effect of the incontinence on the patient's quality of life
5. Factors that affect management (for examples, the patient's mentation, motivation, mobility, and resources)

Patient History

Bowel Function. The interviewer begins by asking the patient to describe his or her past and present bowel function and current problems with bowel control (Fig. 8-6). The interviewer explores with the patient the onset of the incontinence and its duration; this exploration permits the interviewer to differentiate transient incontinence, perhaps related to episodes of diarrhea, from long-standing incontinence. In discussing the onset of incontinence, the interviewer seeks clues to the cause of the incontinence. (For example, the beginning of the incontinence may correspond to the occurrence of a neurologic injury such as cerebrovascular accident or an exacerbation of inflammatory bowel disease.)

The interviewer then asks the patient to describe current patterns of defecation and soiling. The patient is asked about the frequency of controlled (continent) defecation and then asked about the frequency and severity of incontinent episodes. The interviewer must distinguish between the inability to control flatus or the leakage of small amounts of stool (that is, a small smear on the underclothes) and the loss of a bolus of stool several times a day. True incontinence should be differentiated from anal discharge. A spurious incontinence may occur with such conditions as prolapsing hemorrhoids, mucosal prolapse or ectropion, or a keyhole deformity (a gutter formed by posterior midline internal sphincterotomy).[13] In such cases, seepage of fecal-stained mucus and soiling occur but there is no incontinence of solid stool or flatus.

Determining the patient's awareness of the impending incontinence is also helpful. Was the patient aware of impending leakage but unable to prevent it, or was he or she unaware of the imminent incontinence and aware of incontinence only after it occurred? Lack of awareness indicates sensory dysfunction: either a central or a peripheral neuropathy. Awareness with inability to prevent leakage indicates defective sphincter function or inadequate rectal accommodation or both.

The interviewer must also assess the usual consistency of the patient's stool: a sphincter that can hold solid stool may not be competent for liquid stool. Diarrhea is the most common cause of incontinence in patients with normal sphincter mechanisms. Diarrhea may be associated with symptoms of frequency

Name _____ Sex M _____ F _____ Age_____
Duration of incontinence _____
_____

Degree of incontinence
Discharge _____ Soiling _____ Urgency _____ Gas _____ Liquid _____ Solid _____
Bowel habit
Number of bowel movements per day _____
Stool consistency
Watery _____ Loose _____ Formed _____ Hard _____

Frequency of incontinence
Number of episodes per day _____ Number of days of incontinence per week _____
Time of day _____ Time of night _____
Relevant medical history
Number of pregnancies/deliveries _____ Traumatic delivery? _____
History of anorectal surgery _____ Gastrointestinal surgery _____
Trauma to perineum _____ Trauma to spinal cord (level) _____
Neurologic disease _____ Diabetes _____ Radiation therapy _____
Urinary incontinence _____ Impotence _____
Medication for diarrhea _____ Other medications _____
Other illness _____

Fig. 8-6 Form for assessment of patient history. (From MacLeod JH: Endoscopy Rev 5:45, 1988.)

and urgency as well as incontinence. On the other hand, constipation may precipitate incontinence: impacted stool in the rectum causes relaxation of the internal sphincter, and liquified stool can then leak around the fecal mass. (The patient or caregiver is likely to report this leakage as diarrhea.)

In talking with patients, the interviewer must avoid the use of undefined terms such as "diarrhea" and "constipation". The patient should be asked to actually describe the consistency of the stool (for example, watery, runny, mushy, soft, formed, or hard), the volume of stool, and the frequency of the incontinence. The interviewer should realize that many patients with incontinence refer to the incontinence as "diarrhea" and admit to incontinence only on direct questioning. In one study of 76 patients referred for investigation of diarrhea, 38 patients actually had fecal incontinence.[11] Apparently diarrhea is a more socially acceptable symptom.

The patient is also asked about factors that commonly affect stool consistency and volume and frequency of defecation. Factors that commonly affect stool consistency and volume and frequency of defecation include dietary bulk, dietary irritants, fluid intake, past and present use of peristaltic stimulants (laxatives or enemas), medications, physical activity, and emotional status. The interviewer attempts to quantify the patient's usual intake of fluids, dietary bulk, and potential dietary irritants (for example, chocolate or milk products) by asking the patient to describe a typical day's food intake and to identify foods that he or she likes and dislikes. The patient is also asked to describe his or her activity during a typical day. In assessing the patient for possible bowel dependency, the interviewer must ask the patient specific questions regarding past and present use of bowel stimulants (including type of stimulant, frequency of use, and duration of use). Finally, the patient is asked about any change in bowel habits that he or she has observed during emotionally stressful periods. With exploration, patients or caregivers are frequently able to correlate changes in bowel function with one or more of the factors discussed in this paragraph.

After asking the patient to describe the problem of fecal incontinence, the interviewer encourages the patient to describe its effect on his or her life, including the effect on the patient's self-concept and family, social, and sexual relationships, and any changes in the patient's daily activities and routines. The patient is asked to describe his or her current method of management and to identify his or her goals in seeking medical evaluation and treatment.

Focused Review of Systems. After obtaining data regarding the frequency, severity, and effect of fecal incontinence, the interviewer conducts a focused review of systems to elicit clues to the cause of the incontinence (Fig. 8-6). The patient is asked about illness or surgery involving the gastrointestinal tract, since absorption and motility must be normal to deliver formed stool to the rectum at appropriate intervals. History of malabsorption syndromes, inflammatory processes, bowel resection, and anorectal anomalies, injuries, or surgical procedures are all significant. The patient is also asked about genitourinary diseases or disorders; problems with bladder control and, in men, problems with erection or ejaculation suggest impairment of pelvic floor innervation. In women the obstetric history is especially important, since stretch injuries or lacerations are common causes of anorectal denervation and sphincteric damage.[6,15,19] Assessment of the patient's neurologic system is critical, since any disease or disorder of the central or peripheral nervous system can affect pelvic floor innervation and sphincter control (for example, disseminated sclerosis, spinal cord injury, or alterations in mentation). The patient is asked about any chronic illnesses or conditions, such as diabetes. The potential for bowel dysfunction in the patient with diabetes is discussed in Chapter 7.[22]

Finally, the patient is asked about his or her use of prescription and over-the-counter medications; there are a number of medications that can affect stool consistency, bowel motility, mentation, or a combination of these and thus affect continence. Some of the most commonly used medications that can cause diarrhea are antacids that contain magnesium, antibiotics, stool softeners and laxatives, and cholinergic drugs. Anticholinergics, smooth-muscle relaxants, analgesics, and tranquilizers can cause constipation.

Bowel Function Diary

The patient is asked to maintain a diary for 1 to 2 weeks before treatment is begun. In the diary the patient should record time, volume, and consistency of both voluntary (controlled) and involuntary (incontinent) defecation (Fig. 8-7). The patient is asked to maintain such a record throughout the treatment

---

DIARY

Please read the following instructions carefully

For at least one week before Biofeedback is begun, information and observations regarding incontinent episodes need to be entered diligently into the chart. Please continue to enter information until treatment is complete, as it will serve as a reference for your progress. It is important to record successful toilet visits as well as incontinent episodes. Be specific as to the type and degree of the incontinent episode; that is, specify whether gas or stool has escaped and whether it was slight or a "major accident." Also, if it was a stool that has escaped, record whether it was formed or loose. The number and duration of sphincter exercises performed each day should be recorded as well.

To simplify recording, use the following abbreviations:

BM—voluntary bowel movement (successful toilet visit)
ICS—incontinent episode involving *stool*
    either: SL—slight soiling of perineum or underwear
    or   SH—heavily soiled
    or   MA—"major accident"—evacuation in underwear
as well, enter either ES—formed stool
                LS—loose stool
ICG—incontinent episode involving *gas*
SphEx—sphincter exercises

Date	Morning	Afternoon	Evening	Night	Observations

Fig. 8-7   Bowel function diary. (From MacLeod JH: Endoscopy Rev 5:45, 1988.)

program so that progress can be measured; the diary should be reviewed with the patient at each visit. The nurse or the physician or both should stress to the patient the importance of maintaining the diary with as much accuracy as possible because the diary frequently serves as a guide for modification of the treatment program. A simple diary that can be used to assess progress in bowel training programs is shown in Fig. 8-8.

Date and time	Stimulus to evacuation (digital, suppository, or none)	Response (amount and consistency of stool)	Incontinent episodes (time, amount, and type of leakage)

Fig. 8-8   Simple diary of bowel function.

Inspection

Perianal soiling _____   Excoriations _____   Soiling _____

Patulousness _____   Keyhole deformity _____   Wink _____

Straining Perineal descent _____   Sphincter defect _____

            Prolapse _____   Site _____

Digital Examination

Sphincter Resting tone _____   Maximal squeeze   Sphincter defect _____

                                                                  Site _____

Accessory muscle contraction _____

Anorectal angle At rest _____   Contraction _____   Straining _____

Patulousness _____   Closing reflex _____

Posterior traction _____   Bidigital _____   Impaction_____

Anoscopy

Scarring _____   Prolapse of mucosa or hemorrhoids _____

Sigmoidoscopy

Stool consistency _____   Escape of insufflated air _____

Internal intussusception or prolapse _____

Fig. 8-9 Form for physical examination of patient with fecal incontinence. (From MacLeod JH: Endoscopy Rev 5:45, 1988.)

Physical Examination

    The physical examination focuses on the assessment of sphincter integrity and function, rectal vault contents, and the patient's mobility and dexterity (Fig. 8-9).

    Visual Inspection of Anus. The examination begins with a visual inspection of the anal sphincter. The examiner looks for evidence of a divided sphincter, that is, dimples that mark the ends of the divided sphincter or skin folds radiating from the defect. The examiner spreads the buttocks and looks for any gaping of the anus, which may indicate sphincter injury or neurologic impairment (Fig. 8-10). A *gentle* stroke of the perianal area with a pin should elicit a circumferential sphincteric contraction called an anal wink, which is lost if the reflex spinal arc is interrupted at any level. The absence of an anal wink warrants further neurologic examination.

    The patient may be asked to strain while the examiner looks for a bulging of the anus below the level of the most prominent part of the buttocks, the ischial tuberosities; such a finding suggests excessive perineal descent.[6,19] This

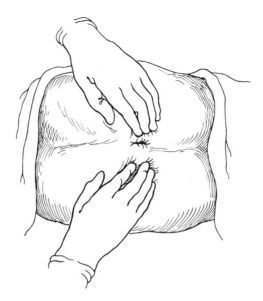

Fig. 8-10 Gentle retraction of perianum may show gaping of anal canal. (From MacLeod JH: A method of proctology, New York, 1979, Harper & Row, Publishers, Inc, p 8.)

finding may indicate neuropathy, either spinal or peripheral. If incontinence is thought to be caused by a neurologic disease or disorder, evaluation by a neurologist is indicated.

Digital Examination of Anus and Rectum. The examiner first assesses the contents of the rectal vault and checks for fecal impaction; sphincter tone at rest and the sphincter's response to voluntary contraction are then assessed.

In evaluating sphincter contractility, the examiner should determine whether the sphincter contracts circumferentially or whether a defect is evident (Fig. 8-11). The examiner then further inserts his or her finger to the top of the sphincter complex in order to assess the anorectal angle and voluntary contraction of the puborectalis (Fig. 8-12).

Determination of normal sphincter response is largely subjective and largely governed by the examiner's experience; however, very little experience is necessary to become familiar with the normal state of sphincter contraction. The normal sphincter complex is in a state of contraction at rest; thus the examining finger is gripped snugly, and voluntary contraction of the normal sphincter is also easily detected. In the patient with deficient sphincter function the sphincter may be lax at rest, and when the patient is instructed to contract the sphincter voluntarily, the examiner may detect little or no contraction.

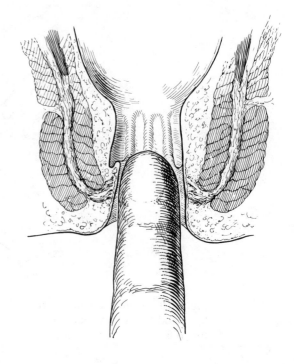

Fig. 8-11 Sphincter tone and integrity is assessed at rest and during contraction. (From MacLeod JH: A method of proctology, New York, 1979, Harper & Row, Publishers, Inc, p 10.)

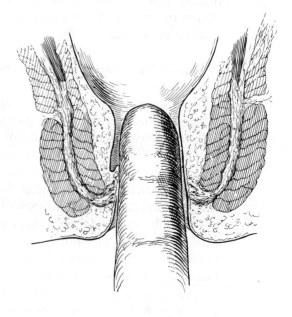

Fig. 8-12 Examining finger is inserted deeper (to middle interphalangeal joint) to assess anorectal angle and tone of puborectalis. (From MacLeod JH: A method of proctology, New York, 1979, Harper & Row, Publishers, Inc, p 10.)

Subtle degrees of patulousness may be detected by gentle posterior traction on the anorectal ring; normally the sphincter continues to close on the finger, but if there is a sphincter deficit, this closure does not occur.[3] Gaps in the muscle are sometimes easier to detect with the two index fingers partly inserted and pulling against each other.

A closing reflex should occur when the examiner's finger is withdrawn; this reflex is normally brisk. If the reflex is defective, the muscle tires rapidly when the finger is inserted and withdrawn several times in succession.

Patient Mobility and Dexterity. The examiner assesses the patient's gait, the time required for position change and ambulation, use of assistive devices, and the patient's ability to manipulate clothing rapidly in preparation for toileting. Any deficits in independent ambulation and toileting must be addressed in a management program.

Laboratory and Radiographic Studies

Laboratory Studies. Laboratory studies may be necessary when the patient's history and physical reveal a disease or disorder of the intestinal tract; for example, diarrhea of unknown origin necessitates further investigation, which may include analysis of stool for the presence of ova and parasites and stool culture and sensitivity tests. Malabsorption syndromes may also necessitate laboratory studies.

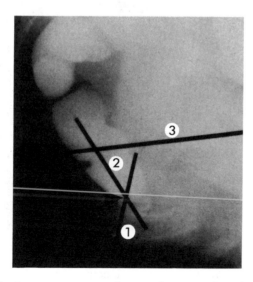

Fig. 8-13 Radiologic measurement of normal anorectal angle. Arrow shows obtuse anorectal angle formed by linear axis of anal canal, *1*, where it intersects axis of rectum, *2*, pubococcygeal line, *3*, is also shown. (From Rosen L et al: Am Fam Physician 33[3]:131, 1986.)

Radiographic Studies. Radiographic studies may be indicated for further investigation of diseases or disorders of the intestinal tract; in addition, certain radiographic studies are used to examine anal continence mechanisms.

Defecography. After the rectum has been filled with barium suspension, the patient is placed on a radiolucent chair and asked to defecate and contract the sphincter while sequential lateral radiographic films are made. Although the study is useful in evaluating the pelvic floor muscle, special equipment is nec-

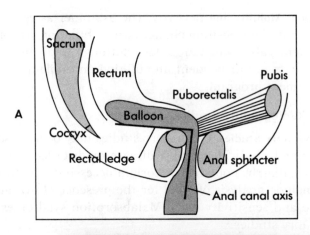

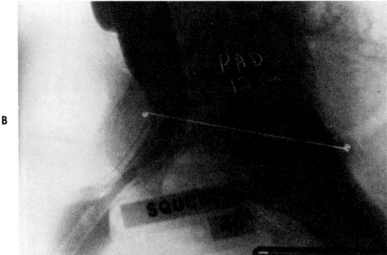

Fig. 8-14 A, Proper measurement of anorectal angle: normal and squeeze. **B,** Sphincterogram showing changes that occur normally when pelvic muscles are squeezed to maintain continence. Anal canal lengthens, anorectal angle sharpens, and puborectalis shortens. (**A** from Lahr CJ: Practical Gastroenterol, 12:27, 1988. **B** from Lahr CJ et al: Dis Colon Rectum 31[5]:349, 1988.)

essary. Defecography displays the anorectal angle and the length of the anal canal and demonstrates perineal descent, if present (Fig. 8-13).[8]

  Balloon sphincterography. Balloon sphincterography provides an evaluation of the external sphincter mechanism of anal canal closure and the production of the anorectal angle by the puborectalis just as manometry does, but the method of balloon sphincterography is much simpler.[10] A cylindrical balloon is placed within the anal canal and rectum and connected by tubing to a bag

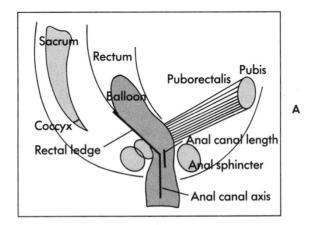

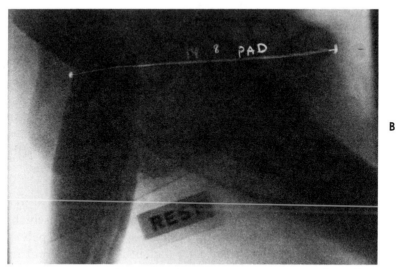

Fig. 8-15   **A,** Squeeze in patient with incontinence. **B,** Sphincterogram of patient with incontinence. Patient is at rest with hips slightly flexed. Weakening of sphincter and puborectalis muscles produces flatter angle and shorter anal canal. (**A** from Lahr CJ: Practical Gastroenterol, 12:27, 1988. **B** from Lahr CJ et al: Dis Colon Rectum 31[5]:350, 1988.)

of radiopaque dye. The pressure in the balloon corresponds to the height of the fluid in the bag and can be increased or decreased by raising or lowering the bag (Fig. 8-14). The shape of the flexible, dye-filled balloon within the anal canal and rectum is visualized by fluoroscopy or plain films or both during voluntary contraction and relaxation of the external sphincter and puborectalis; the resting and maximum squeeze pressures are measured and recorded, as are the length of the anal canal and the degree of perineal descent (Fig. 8-15).

A disposable kit for balloon sphincterography is available commercially at a reasonable cost, and the procedure can be performed in any radiology department. However, the accuracy and reliability of this method have been questioned recently.[7]

Ultrasonography. The relatively new procedure of ultrasonography is able to provide early evidence of abnormalities of the pelvic floor and the anorectal angle. The procedure is the same as that used in balloon sphincterography except that ultrasound is used in place of fluoroscopy and radiographs; the use of ultrasound eliminates concern regarding exposure to radiation (Fig. 8-16).[16]

Studies of Anorectal Physiology

The history and physical examination are by far the most important measures in the evaluation of the patient with incontinence.[3] Other studies rarely influence the physician's decision for or against surgery.

However, further testing sometimes helps the examiner determine which component of continence is affected, that is, sensory function, motor function, or rectal capacity and compliance.

For many years investigators "attacked" their "unfortunate" patients with tubes, balloons, and needle electrodes, but the anorectum was slow to reveal its secrets. Recently, however, an information explosion related to the physiology of the anorectum has occurred. Several hospitals, especially those in major teaching centers, have established laboratories for the study of manometry, electromyography, and defecography, both for research purposes and as methods of clinical evaluation. These studies have contributed greatly to our understanding of the pathophysiology of incontinence.

Sensory Function. Normal sensory function is critical to continence; sensory function alerts the individual to rectal distention, which is the stimulus to voluntary contraction of the external sphincter and pelvic floor musculature. The test for sensitivity to rectal distention is simple but important; it is most valuable when performed before any proposed sphincter repair because sphincter repair in the individual with impaired sensitivity is not likely to correct the incontinence. The examiner should be particularly suspicious of impaired sensitivity in the patient with incontinence who has normal sphincter tone.

The sensory threshold is the smallest volume of rectal distention sensed by

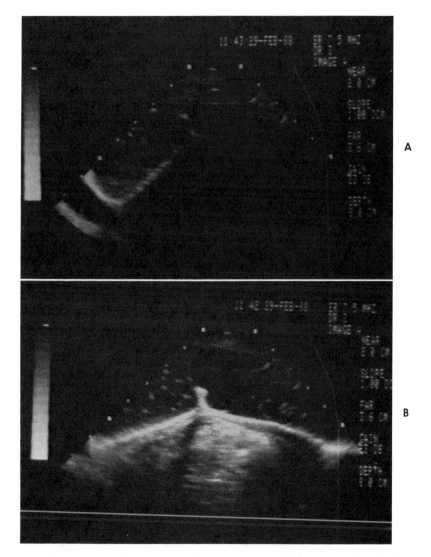

Fig. 8-16   Ultrasonographic images of anorectum. **A,** With contraction. **B,** At rest. (From Pittman JS, Benson JT, and Sumners JE: Dis Colon Rectum 33:477, 1990.)

the patient and is normally 15 ml. Sensory threshold is measured by inflating an intrarectal balloon with air until the patient senses distention.

Normally the patient is aware of the distention in less than 2 seconds.[1] A few patients have a delayed response to rectal distention because they respond to the wrong stimulus; that is, they do not contract the sphincter until they feel the sphincter being stretched by the full rectum.

Patients may have impaired sensory function with or without an associated motor deficit. Some patients are able to contract the external sphincter on command but do not perceive rectal distention and are therefore deprived of the appropriate warning signal (Table 8-2).[12]

Motor Function. Normal sphincter function requires intact and normally innervated musculature and can be evaluated by anorectal manometry and electromyography.

Anorectal manometry. Anorectal manometry measures the resting tone of the internal sphincter, the contractility of the external sphincter, and the functional length of the anal canal.[2,3] All methods of anorectal manometry involve the insertion of a catheter, which is connected to a transducer and a recorder or computer, but the different methods have little else in common. (The examiner must be aware that the presence of a catheter, even of narrow caliber, constitutes an artifact and that catheters of different diameters affect the readings to varying extents.)

The intra-anal catheter may be closed, as in Schuster's method.[18] This method involves the use of a probe with three balloons: an intrarectal balloon, which can be inflated to cause rectal distention, a proximal intra-anal balloon, which records internal sphincter contraction and relaxation, and a distal intra-anal balloon, which records external sphincter contraction and relaxation (Fig. 8-17).

In other systems, the intra-anal balloon is open either at its end or through side openings (the number and size of side openings are variable); the open catheter is perfused with water. The rate of infusion must be rapid enough to reflect anal pressure changes promptly but not so rapid that it produces an excessive accumulation of fluid in the rectum.

Since the anal sphincter exerts different pressures at different points along its axis, a longitudinal profile is desirable. This profile of the anal sphincter both at rest and during contraction is obtained by withdrawing the catheter. The catheter may be withdrawn by station pull-out (that is, withdrawal is stopped at intervals such as 1 cm, and pressure is measured at each interval) or by continuous pull-out (that is, the catheter is withdrawn by a mechanical pulling device). In either method, withdrawal of the catheter must be completed within 1 minute, since the sphincter can be contracted maximally for only that long.[2]

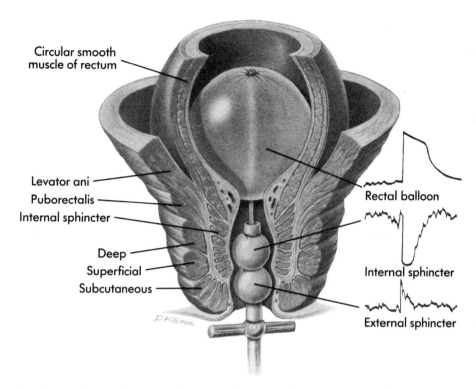

Circular smooth
muscle of rectum

Levator ani
Puborectalis
Internal sphincter

Deep
Superficial
Subcutaneous

Rectal balloon

Internal sphincter

External sphincter

Fig. 8-17 Coronal section of anus and rectum showing anorectal musculature. Three-balloon system is located in rectal ampulla, region of internal sphincter, and external sphincter, respectively. Tracings indicate pressure changes for each balloon after distention of balloon in rectum. (From Rosen L et al: Am Fam Physician 33[3]:130, 1986.)

Manometric resting and contractile pressures are decreased in cases of sphincter laceration and denervation and during a reflex reaction to rectal distention (for example, in cases of fecal impaction). These pressures are increased in cases of anal fissure and in some patients with hemorrhoids.

The many methods of anorectal manometry render comparison between centers difficult if not impossible. However, all methods should demonstrate anal canal pressures, both resting pressure and maximum squeeze pressure, as well as the rectoanal, or rectosphincteric, reflex (that is, relaxation of the internal sphincter and contraction of the external sphincter in response to balloon distention of the rectum).[2]

Sphincter electromyography. Electrodes are used in electromyography to measure the activity of the external sphincter muscle. The placement of the needle electrodes has been painful in the past; the advent of fine, hairlike wire electrodes has made the procedure more acceptable recently. The electrodes are inserted into the puborectalis and external sphincter; no anesthesia is given. The patient is then encouraged to contract the sphincter maximally, and the degree of response is evaluated. One limitation of electromyography is that abnormal potentials may be difficult to detect because the external sphincter is an atypical striated muscle; that is, it maintains tonus even when it is not voluntarily contracted.

Electromyography may be used to help identify the location of the external sphincter when the normal anatomy has been disrupted, as in cases of congenital anomaly or trauma.[23] A more recent development, single-fiber electromyography, can identify muscle denervation and give an estimate of its degree.[6,19]

Reservoir Function. As previously discussed, continence beyond the period of maximal sphincter contraction depends on the rectum's ability to accommodate the fecal mass; the capacity and compliance of the rectum must be adequate. The rectum's ability to serve as a reservoir can be assessed by inserting a large-capacity balloon such as a finger cot or a condom well into the rectum; the balloon is tied to the end of a length of polyethylene tubing, which is connected to a three-way stopcock and a 50 cc syringe. The balloon is then inflated in 50 cc increments, and rectal accommodation is determined (Table 8-3).

Quantification (Severity) Study. In the assessment of the patient with fecal incontinence it is helpful to objectively determine the degree, or severity, of the fecal incontinence. The saline continence test is a simple method of quantifying the incontinence and monitoring the response to treatment.[17]

A funnel and a graduated cylinder are placed beneath the seat of a toilet, and the patient is seated on the commode. A saline solution is run into the rectum through a length of polyethylene tubing at the rate of 60 ml/min for 25 minutes. The first leak (greater than 10 ml) and the total retained volume are measured. A volume of 1500 ml is usually retained in continent individuals,

Table 8-3 Rectal reservoir

Rectal accommodation	Normal value (cc)
Initial sensation (sensory threshold)	15
Constant volume (substantial feeling of fullness)	150
Maximum tolerated volume (limit of tolerance or balloon expelled)	250 to 400

From MacLeod JH: Endoscopy Rev 5:45, 1988.

whereas patients with incontinence almost invariably have leakage when approximately 500 ml has been instilled.

This quantification study reliably discriminates between continence and incontinence and provides an overall measure of the degree of continence or incontinence. The result varies with the strength of the external sphincter, the degree of rectal compliance, and the motivation of the patient.

Psychosocial Assessment

As previously discussed, the objective of assessment is to develop a treatment plan that appropriately addresses the pathophysiologic mechanisms and is acceptable to and manageable for the patient or caregiver. Therefore the patient's mentation and ability to participate in a treatment plan, as well as the patient's motivation, must be assessed: cognitive dysfunction or lack of motivation can sabotage the best treatment plans. If the patient is alert, oriented, and motivated, all diagnostic results should be shared with him or her, and a treatment plan should be jointly established. If the patient's mentation or motivation do not support such an effort, the practitioner must work with the caregiver to establish a treatment plan that meets the caregiver's goals and is manageable. In addition, resources available to the patient or caregiver must be evaluated, including the financial resources and the persons available to support the treatment plan.

Table 8-4   Methods used to assess fecal incontinence*

Component	Method
SENSORY	
Anal	Touch
Rectal	Balloon
MOTOR	
External sphincter and puborectalis	Manometry
	Radiology
	Electromyography
RESERVOIR	
Rectal capacity and compliance	Radiology
	Balloon
Colon capacity and motility	Colonoscopy or barium enema or both
	Transit studies

*To be used in addition to history and examination.
From MacLeod JH: Fecal incontinence: Endoscopy Rev 5:45, 1988.

SUMMARY

Accurate and comprehensive assessment is the critical first component of effective management for the patient with fecal incontinence. During assessment the practitioner seeks to identify causative factors, determine which continence mechanisms are involved, evaluate the severity of the incontinence and its impact on the patient's life, and explore factors that may affect the treatment plan.

The history and physical remain the mainstays in the assessment of fecal incontinence. Advances in anorectal physiology testing are increasing our ability to determine accurately which components of continence are impaired; thus we are able to treat the incontinence more effectively. Table 8-4 summarizes methods currently used to assess fecal incontinence.

Finally, the practitioner must always remember that assessment focuses on the patient with incontinence, not the incontinence itself. Thus a comprehensive assessment includes evaluation of the effect of incontinence on the patient and his or her life-style, and the patient's goals are considered when the treatment plan is being determined.

SELF-EVALUATION

QUESTIONS

1. Differentiate between continence at rest and continence in the presence of rectal distention in terms of internal and external sphincter function.
2. Explain what is meant by the statement, "Continence is relative, not 'all or none.'"
3. Identify three objectives of the assessment of the patient with fecal incontinence.
4. Identify data to be included in an initial bowel history for the patient with fecal incontinence.
5. Explain the relationship between diarrhea and fecal incontinence, and the implications for the assessment of patients with diarrhea.
6. Identify information to be gathered in a focused systems review for the patient with fecal incontinence.
7. Identify data to be included in a bowel function diary.
8. Identify data that the nurse can obtain from a visual and digital examination of the anus and rectum.
9. Identify two radiographic studies that specifically assess structures and functions related to fecal continence.
10. Explain the role of anorectal physiology studies in the evaluation of the patient with fecal incontinence.
11. Match the anorectal study to the component of the continence mechanism that it evaluates:
    a. Intrarectal balloon or air inflation study
    b. Electromyography
    c. Anorectal manometry
    d. Balloon reservoir study
    e. Balloon sphincterography
    1. Motor
    2. Sensory
    3. Rectal capacity and compliance
12. Normal sensory threshold for rectal distention is approximately:
    a. 300 ml
    b. 100 ml
    c. 15 ml
    d. 2 ml
13. Describe normal results of anorectal manometry in terms of:
    a. Internal sphincter response
    b. External sphincter response
14. Normal rectal capacity (maximum retained volume as measured by the reservoir study) is approximately:
    a. 100 to 150 ml
    b. 150 to 250 ml

       c. 250 to 400 ml

       d. 500 ml

15. Explain the importance of the patient's mentation and motivation and the resources of the patient or caregiver in the development of an appropriate treatment plan.

SELF-EVALUATION

ANSWERS

1. Continence at rest is maintained primarily by the internal sphincter, which is contracted maximally. Continence in the presence of rectal distention is maintained primarily by external sphincter contraction, which increases the anal canal pressure until the peristaltic wave subsides and the rectum stretches to accommodate the fecal mass. The internal sphincter relaxes in response to rectal distention.

2. Many factors affect fecal continence. Impairment of one factor may not result in incontinence unless the impairment is severe. For example, the person with intact sensation and normal sphincter function may be able to maintain continence except when the volume of stool is so large that it overwhelms the rectum's capacity to serve as a reservoir. In managing the patient with incontinence, the nurse should remember that disruption of one continence mechanism can sometimes be compensated for, if other mechanisms remain intact. For example, continence in the patient with impaired sphincter function may be maintained, if appropriate stool volume and consistency are maintained.

3. **a.** To identify the cause of the incontinence
   b. To determine which component of the continence mechanism is affected (sensory, motor, or reservoir)
   c. To determine the degree, or severity, of the incontinence
   d. To evaluate the effect of the incontinence on the patient's quality of life
   e. To explore factors that affect management

4. **a.** Onset and duration of the incontinence
   b. Patterns of defecation and soiling
   c. Sensation or awareness of impending incontinence
   d. Usual stool consistency, volume, and frequency
   e. Factors that affect stool consistency and volume (diet, fluids, and medications)
   f. Effect of incontinence on the patient's self-esteem, relationships, and life-style

5. The patient with fecal incontinence may seek medical advice because of diarrhea; therefore, patients with diarrhea should be carefully assessed for fecal incontinence.

   Acute or chronic diarrhea may overwhelm continence mechanisms and precipitate diarrhea; therefore, management of the patient with diarrhea and fecal incontinence should focus initially on correction of the diarrhea.

   Fecal impaction can result in a secondary diarrhea; therefore, patients with diarrhea should be evaluated for fecal impaction.

6. **a.** Gastrointestinal system: resections, malabsorption syndromes, inflammatory processes, and anorectal anomalies, injuries, or surgical procedures

   b. Genitourinary system: problems with bladder control
   Men: sexual dysfunction
   Women: obstetric history, including the number of pregnancies and deliveries, difficult deliveries, and injuries

   c. Neurologic system: any lesion, disease, or condition that affects the function of the central or peripheral nervous system

   d. Chronic illnesses, for example, diabetes

   e. Medication profile (use of any drugs that affect the gastrointestinal tract, the central or autonomic nervous system, or muscle function)

7. **a.** Voluntary (controlled) bowel movements

   b. Incontinent episodes (type and volume of leakage and time of leakage)

8. **a.** Any visual evidence of a divided sphincter (dimples or skin folds) or sphincter dysfunction (gaping of the anus when the buttocks are spread or loss of the anal wink in response to a gentle pin stroke)

   b. Presence or absence of fecal impaction

   c. Sphincter tone at rest

   d. Patient's ability to voluntarily contract sphincter

9. **a.** Defecography

   b. Balloon sphincterography

10. Anorectal physiology studies determine which components of the continence mechanism are impaired (that is, sensory, motor, or reservoir)

11. **a.** 2. Sensory

    b. 1. Motor

    c. 1. Motor

    d. 3. Rectal capacity and compliance

    e. 1. Motor

12. **c.** 15 ml

13. **a.** The internal sphincter should show contraction during rectal filling and should relax when rectal distention occurs.

    b. The external sphincter should contract when the rectum is distended.

14. **c.** 250 to 400 ml

15. The treatment plan must be carried out by the patient or caregiver or both; therefore the plan must be compatible with their goals, abilities, and resources.

REFERENCES

1. Buser WD and Miner PB: Delayed rectal sensation with fecal incontinence, Gastroenterology 91:1186, 1986.
2. Coller J: Clinical application of anorectal manometry, Surg Clin North Am 16:17, 1987.
3. Corman ML: Colon and rectal surgery, ed 2, Philadelphia, 1989, JB Lippincott Co.
4. Dalley AF: The riddle of the sphincters: the morphophysiology of the anorectal mechanism reviewed, Am Surg 53:298, 1987.
5. Duthie HL and Cairns FW: The sensory nerve endings and sensation in the anal region of man, Br J Surg 47:585, 1960.
6. Henry MM, Parks AG, and Swash M: The pelvic floor musculature in the descending perineum syndrome, Br J Surg 69:470, 1982.
7. Keighley MRB et al: Anorectal physiology measurement: report of a working party, Br J Surg 76:356, 1989.
8. Kuijpers HC and Strijk SP: Diagnosis of disturbances of continence and defecation, Dis Colon Rectum 27:658, 1984.
9. Lahr CJ et al: Balloon topography, a simple method of evaluating anal function, Dis Colon Rectum 29:1, 1986.
10. Lane RH and Parks AG: Function of the anal sphincters following colo-anal anastomosis, Br J Surg 64:596, 1977.
11. Leigh RJ and Turnberg LA: Faecal incontinence: the unvoiced symptom, Lancet 1:1349, 1982.
12. Lubowski DZ and Nicholls RJ: Faecal incontinence associated with reduced pelvic sensation, Br J Surg 75:1086, 1989.
13. Mazier WP: Keyhole deformity: fact and fiction, Dis Colon Rectum 28:8, 1985.
14. Miller R et al: Anorectal sampling: a comparison of normal and incontinent patients, Br J Surg 75:44, 1988.
15. Parks AG: Anorectal incontinence, Proc R Soc Med 68:681, 1975.
16. Pittman JS, Benson JT, and Sumners JE: Physiologic evaluation of the anorectum, a new ultrasound technique, Dis Colon Rectum 33:476, 1990.
17. Read NW et al: A clinical study of patients with fecal incontinence and diarrhea, Gastroenterology 76:747, 1979.
18. Schuster MM: Clinical applications of rectosphincteric manometry, Endoscopy Rev 2:68, 1985.
19. Swash M: Anorectal incontinence: electrophysiological tests, Br J Surg 72[Suppl]:14, 1985.
20. Thomson JPS: Anal sphincter incompetence. In Russell RGD, ed: Recent advances in surgery, London, 1986, Churchill Livingstone, Inc.
21. Wald A: Fecal incontinence: effective nonsurgical treatments, Postgrad Med 80:123, 1986.
22. Wald A and Tunuguntla AK: Anorectal sensorimotor dysfunction in fecal incontinence and diabetes mellitus, N Engl J Med 310:1282, 1984.
23. Waylonis GD and Powers JJ: Clinical application of anal sphincter electromyography, Surg Clin North Am 52:807, 1972.

9 Management of Fecal Incontinence

ALICE BASCH
LINDA JENSEN

OBJECTIVES

1. Identify environmental adaptations that may facilitate continence in the older or less mobile individual.

2. Identify common causes of chronic diarrhea.

3. Explain the purpose and procedure for an elimination diet.

4. Identify at least two clinical conditions that can result in malabsorption and diarrhea.

5. Identify indications for the use of elemental diets in the management of malabsorption and diarrhea.

6. Identify common causes of acute diarrhea and the implications for nursing assessment and management.

7. Explain why the enterally fed patient is at risk for diarrhea, and identify appropriate nursing interventions for this patient.

8. Describe measures that may be employed to control diarrhea until the underlying cause can be corrected.

9. Identify indications for the use of external fecal collection devices.

10. Identify potential adverse reactions associated with the use of internal fecal drainage systems and implications for nursing care.

11. Describe appropriate measures for the prevention and management of skin breakdown in the patient with diarrhea or fecal incontinence or both.

12. Describe the usual appearance and appropriate treatment of a fungal rash.

13. Identify the initial goal of treatment in management of the patient with chronic constipation.

14. Identify at least two methods of providing adequate bulk for the patient with constipation.

15. Identify candidates for bowel training programs, and outline the components of a successful bowel training program.

16. Compare and contrast the various methods of stimulating rectal evacuation, that is, digital stimulation, suppositories, mini-enemas, and enemas.

17. Explain the concept and procedure for sensory reeducation.

18. Identify patients who may benefit from sphincter retraining.

19. Explain the potential benefit of biofeedback therapy in a sphincter retraining program.

20. Identify candidates for sphincter repair surgery.

21. Describe the gracilis muscle transfer procedure, including indications, procedure, and results.

As discussed in previous chapters, fecal continence depends on normal stool consistency and volume, adequate rectal capacity and compliance, intact sensory function, and normal sphincteric function. Alterations in any of these factors can result in bowel dysfunction and fecal incontinence. Mobility and environmental factors may also affect the individual's ability to maintain continence.

Fecal incontinence in both ambulatory and nonambulatory persons is a concern for all health care providers. Management of these individuals should encompass measures to restore continence and measures to control symptoms. Measures to restore continence may include environmental manipulation, dietary alterations, bowel training programs, sensory reeducation, sphincter training exercises, medications, and surgical procedures to correct an underlying defect. Symptom control measures may include fecal containment devices, skin protection, and odor control. The nurse plays a key role in restoration of continence and control of symptoms and in support and education for the patient and family.

ENVIRONMENTAL MANIPULATION

Manipulation of the environment to promote continence is a basic nursing responsibility but one that is frequently overlooked: often health care providers assume that a person past a certain age or with a certain disease or disability will have incontinence. By maintaining a positive attitude related to achieving continence and providing an environment that promotes independence, nurses may help the patient achieve continence.

Recommendations for the ambulatory patient include the following:

1. Bed and chairs at an appropriate height for independent entry and exit
2. Bed and chairs near the bathroom or commode
3. Appropriate walking aids (cane, tripod, or walker)
4. Bathroom doors large enough to accommodate walkers or wheelchairs
5. Adequate numbers of toilets or commodes in large facilities
6. Side rails at the toilet and on the walls
7. Clear markings to bathrooms; lighted hall or night lights
8. Easily manipulated door locks
9. Clothing that facilitates access for toileting (for example, elastic waist bands, snap or Velcro closures, dresses rather than slacks for women)

Recommendations for the nonambulatory patient include the following:

1. Call button or bell within easy reach
2. Clean bedpan within easy reach

MEASURES TO NORMALIZE STOOL CONSISTENCY AND VOLUME

Alterations in stool consistency and volume frequently contribute to the development of fecal incontinence. These factors should be assessed in an initial evaluation of the person with incontinence, and the cause(s) of any abnormality should be determined. Common causes of altered stool consistency and volume are discussed in the following paragraphs, and appropriate interventions are presented.

Chronic Diarrhea

Diarrhea can occur as either an acute or a chronic condition. Chronic diarrhea is likely to result from dietary intolerance, malabsorption conditions, or chronic intestinal conditions that result in motility changes.

Dietary Intolerance. Dietary intolerance can often be detected through an assessment of dietary intake that is correlated with fecal output. The diet and stool history may help identify foods that are poorly tolerated; all foods and fluids (types and amounts) that the patient ingests during 1 week are documented, and the time, volume, and consistency of bowel movements during the same period are also documented (Fig. 9-1). Patients or caregivers should be instructed to include in the diet history such things as sugar, cream, butter, and spices that are added to foods. Poorly tolerated foods are then eliminated from the diet.

Time	Food	Amount	Stool pattern
7:00 AM	Coffee with sugar	2 cups	
	Toast with butter and jam	1 slice	
10:30 AM	Coffee	1 cup	Loose stool
12:15 PM	Ham and cheese sandwich on white bread	1	
	Potato chips	Bag (1 oz)	
	Chocolate chip cookies	2	
	Coffee with sugar	1 cup	Loose stool
2:30 PM	Diet Coke	8 oz	
6:00 PM	White wine	4 oz	
	Pretzels	10 small	
7:00 PM	Roast turkey	3 oz	
	Gravy	2 tbsp	
	Cranberry sauce	½ cup	
	Green beans	½ cup	
	Biscuit with butter	1 small	
	Green salad with blue cheese	3 tbsp	
	Chocolate cake	Medium slice	
	Coffee with sugar	1 cup	Loose stool

Fig. 9-1 Sample diet and stool history.

Elimination diet. A structured elimination diet that is developed in consultation with a registered dietitian is another method used to determine food intolerance.[24] Foods that are known to frequently cause diarrhea (Table 9-1) and any suspect foods (identified by the diet and stool history) are eliminated from the initial diet. If no improvement is found after the patient has followed the initial elimination diet for 2 weeks, a more restricted diet that further eliminates possible offending foods is tried. If improvement is seen with an elimination diet, eliminated foods are reintroduced by adding one food item to the diet about every 3 days. Foods that cause exacerbation of symptoms can be isolated and restricted or eliminated as needed. For this type of dietary manipulation the services of a registered dietitian are helpful; a computer software program (Food Processor II) developed by the Elizabeth Stewart Hands Associates (ESHA) Research Company of Salem, Oregon, is also available.

Lactose intolerance. Some foods cause diarrhea because of a deficiency in the production or utilization of a specific enzyme. Lactose intolerance, for example, results from lactase deficiency.[3,24] Lactose is a sugar found in milk and milk

Table 9-1 Foods that alter stool consistency

Food	Loosens stool	Thickens stool	Comment
Additives			
Nutmeg	X		
Sorbitol	X		Causes flatulence and abdominal distention
Caffeine	X		Increases gastrointestinal motility
Fiber		X	Initially may cause increased gas or diarrhea or both
Bran; dried apricots; dried beans; figs; prunes; rye; winter squash			
Fruits			
Apples		X	Absorbs fluids; decreases motility
Bananas		X	
Milk products	X	X	With lactose intolerance, loosens; otherwise, may thicken
Cottage cheese; processed cheese			
Yogurt; buttermilk			Restores bowel flora
Meat	X		With intolerance
Pork; beef			
Potatoes	X		With intolerance
Wheat	X		With intolerance

products. In the individual with lactase deficiency, the sugar is incompletely digested; incomplete digestion of sugar results in an osmotic diarrhea and increased gas production. When lactose cannot be completely eliminated from the patient's diet, live acidophilus culture can be added to the diet. This culture converts the sugar into glucose and galactose, which the body is better able to tolerate. Soy products and goat's milk may also be better tolerated by the individual with lactase deficiency, and some individuals with lactase deficiency may be able to tolerate small amounts of processed or cultured milk products such as American cheese, cottage cheese, and yogurt.

Celiac disease. A specific intolerance occurs in celiac disease, or nontropical sprue.[3,31,49,51] The offending substance in celiac disease, gluten, is found in a variety of foods such as wheat, rye, oat, barley, yeast, malted milk, Postum, commercially prepared meats (sausage, frankfurters, luncheon meats), and some salad dressings. Even small amounts of gluten can cause severe diarrhea and steatorrhea in individuals with this disease. Some people with celiac disease also have lactose intolerance. A strict, gluten-free diet is the only treatment for individuals with celiac disease. Health food stores and many large grocery stores now stock packaged foods that are gluten free. Such foods can also be ordered from several mail-order companies.

Caffeine. Some foods may alter stool consistency by affecting metabolism or motility. Caffeine, for example, has been known to cause diarrhea in some individuals. Effects of caffeine on the gastrointestinal system include increased production of gastric acid and pepsin and increased intestinal peristalsis.[33] Coffee, tea, cola, and chocolate are the most common sources of caffeine; it is also found in over-the-counter stimulants, analgesics, cold preparations, and certain prescription drugs. As with other types of food intolerance, the reduction or elimination of caffeine may be the best approach.

Alcohol. Alcohol can also induce diarrhea, especially when consumed in large quantities.[31] Reduced production of intestinal enzymes, pancreatic insufficiency, vitamin deficiencies, and hypermotility may be seen in patients who consume large quantities of alcohol. Reduction or elimination of alcohol consumption is the obvious treatment in such cases.

Malabsorption Syndromes

Surgical alterations in intestinal tract. Disease or surgical resection of certain intestinal segments may result in malabsorption syndromes and diarrhea. For example, pancreatic disease or resection of the terminal ileum may interfere with the digestion and absorption of fat, which can result in steatorrhea and weight loss. A fat-restricted diet supplemented with medium-chain triglycerides (Portagen or MCT oil, Mead Johnson & Co., Evansville, Ind.) provides essential fatty acids, promotes absorption of fat-soluble vitamins, and reduces diarrhea.

Another surgical alteration that results in diarrhea is the removal of the pylorus.[28,31] The flow of hyperosmolar substances into the small intestine produces an isosmotic intestinal content approximately 20 to 30 minutes after a meal. The most effective treatment appears to be frequent, small meals that are low in starch and sugar. The consumption of fluids during meals should be avoided. Anticholinergic drugs may also be of benefit, since they slow peristalsis.

Radiation injury to bowel. Radiation injury to the bowel may induce a malabsorption syndrome that results in diarrhea. Mucosal injury may occur during the period of radiation therapy, or the injury may become evident several years after radiation therapy. Low-residue diets may be of benefit for patients who are receiving radiation treatments, especially for those at particular risk for injury (for example, patients receiving abdominal radiation therapy who also have diabetes, hypertension, thin physiques, or bowel adhesions, and patients receiving chemotherapy and abdominal radiation therapy concurrently). Gluten-free, lactose-free, and low-fat diets may be of benefit to patients who have radiation injury to the bowel.[8]

Inflammatory bowel disease. Malabsorption and chronic diarrhea are common results of inflammatory bowel disease.[2,6,26,31,42] Although dietary manipulation is controversial in the management of these diseases, several approaches have been suggested. Lactose, fructose, and sorbitol may exacerbate diarrhea, and some practitioners recommend elimination or limited intake of these substances. Avoidance of roughage, fruit juices, and cruciferous vegetables has also been recommended. Carbohydrate intake may contribute to diarrhea in patients with total colitis, although there appears to be little relationship between carbohydrate intake and diarrhea in patients with distal colitis.[42] A yeast-free diet has been suggested by holistic health care practitioners.[4,20] Low-fat, low-oxalate diets after ileal resection have also been suggested; oxalate is found in green beans, beets, spinach, sweet potatoes, plums, raspberries, almonds, cashew nuts, chocolate, cocoa, and tea.[6] Because the role of diet in the control of inflammatory bowel disease has yet to be clarified, the best approach may be to allow the individual to regulate his or her own diet according to symptoms.

Treatment. In cases of severe malabsorption and diarrhea, dietary modifications alone may not be sufficient to control diarrhea and provide essential nutrients.[31,37a] These patients may require the elimination of all prepared foods and the use of a predigested (elemental) diet that contains 1-amino acids, medium-chain triglycerides, simple sugars, vitamins, and minerals. Examples of prepared elemental diets include Vivonex HN (Norwich-Eaton Pharmaceuticals, Norwich, N.Y.), Flexical (Mead Johnson & Co., Evansville, Ind.), and Vital HN (Ross Laboratories, Columbus, Ohio). The use of medications, as discussed later in this chapter, may also be necessary to control the diarrhea. Total parenteral nutrition (TPN) may be necessary in cases of severe malabsorption syndrome that do not respond to lesser measures.[38,45]

Acute Diarrhea

During an acute episode of diarrhea, incontinence may result.[31] Common causes of acute diarrhea include unrecognized impaction, viral or bacterial gastroenteritis, intestinal candidiasis, and enteral feedings, especially in the patient who is severely malnourished or who has received nothing by mouth for several days.

Fecal Impaction. Overflow incontinence with watery diarrhea is often a symptom of bowel impaction. If the impaction is unrecognized and antidiarrheal agents that further decrease bowel motility are used, serious problems may occur. Any patient at risk for constipation or impaction should be placed on a bowel management program (as discussed later in this chapter), including patients who are receiving certain chemotherapeutic agents or narcotics, patients with reduced mobility, and patients with limited oral intake.[5] If sudden, watery diarrhea should develop in a patient who is at risk for constipation or impaction, an evaluation for impaction should be performed immediately.

Gastroenteritis. Gastroenteritis is a common cause of diarrhea and incontinence. Immunocompromised patients (for example, patients receiving cancer treatment or steroids, malnourished patients, and patients with the human immunodeficiency virus) are at particular risk for bacterial or viral diarrhea. Common causative organisms include *Clostridium difficile, Shigella, Salmonella, Mycobacterium avium intracellulare,* invasive *Escherichia coli,* and *Giardia.*[31,39] Patients who are receiving organ and bone marrow transplants are also at increased risk for gastroenteritis that results from graft-versus-host disease (GVHD). A five-phase management program has been developed by Gauvreau et al.[25] for patients with gastroenteritis resulting from GVHD. A stool culture should be performed for any patient with diarrhea of undetermined origin to rule out the possibility of an infectious process. Treatment based on the results of culture and sensitivity tests should then be initiated, and measures should be taken to control the diarrhea as necessary.

Fungal Superinfection. Aggressive antibiotic therapy can destroy the normal balance of organisms in the intestine and has the potential to cause a fungal superinfection that results in diarrhea. In some settings patients are placed on preventive protocols that include lactobacillus products (Lactinex) or dairy products that contain bacterial cultures (for example, buttermilk or yogurt). When unexplained diarrhea develops in a patient who is receiving antibiotic therapy, the use of antifungal agents should be considered.

Enteral Feedings. Enteral feedings are commonly associated with diarrhea and incontinence. Although the diarrhea is usually attributed to the formula itself, diarrhea is more commonly caused by an underlying malnutrition that results in edema of the gut wall and malabsorption. (An albumin level of less than 2.8/100 ml is often associated with edema.) Malabsorption and diarrhea associated with enteral feedings may also be caused by atrophy of the intestinal villi and the loss of intestinal border enzymes, which result in decreased absorptive surface and capacity.[10,39,47]

Interventions to prevent or control diarrhea in the enterally fed patient can be initiated by the nurse. Formulas should be isotonic, and feedings should be instituted at a slow rate such as 50 ml/hr and gradually advanced. Formulas that contain bulk agents are often recommended. (Bulk agents absorb fluid in the stool, thus normalizing stool consistency.) Antidiarrheal agents may also be necessary during the adaptation phase (until atrophy of the villi is reversed and bowel wall edema is resolved).[10,38] The cessation of feeding in response to diarrhea is one intervention that is not recommended. The underlying causes of the diarrhea (malnutrition with atrophy of villi and bowel wall edema) can be corrected only by providing nutritional support and stimulating the gut.

To prevent bacterial overgrowth in the feeding bag and tubing, routine care and cleaning of the equipment should be strictly performed. Tubing and bags should be replaced daily. For the home care patient who has a dishwasher, hard plastic containers are recommended, since dishwashers render the equipment clean enough to be reused.

Symptom Control Measures. In addition to determining and correcting the underlying reasons for diarrhea, general measures can be used to control symptoms in any individual with diarrhea, including measures to improve stool consistency and reduce volume (bulk agents, constipating diets, and antidiarrheal medications), fluid and electrolyte replacement, and measures to contain stool and protect the skin.

Measures to improve stool consistency

DIETARY MEASURES

Constipating diets or bulk agents that thicken the stool and reduce volume can be used to control diarrhea and fecal incontinence.[12,27] Foods that may help thicken stool include rice, bananas, apples or unfiltered apple juice, yogurt, cheese, marshmallows, and some wheat products. These foods reduce diarrhea by absorbing fluid from the stool. Pectin, which is found in fruits such as apples, is a water-soluble fiber that has a water-binding effect and also tends to reduce gastric emptying.[35] Bulk agents may also be recommended to thicken stool; they work by absorbing fluid in the bowel. A bulk product such as psyllium acts to reduce watery stools and slow transit time.[12,27,37] The recommended dosage for psyllium seed derivatives is 1 to 3 tbsp daily in water or juice. Newer psyllium products are more palatable because of flavorings and are available in different forms (for example, tablet, wafer, and cereal forms). Nongelling bulk agents are also available.

PHARMACOLOGIC MEASURES

The use of pharmacologic agents that reduce diarrhea is often necessary to relieve fecal incontinence. Medications may be used either to achieve appropriate stool consistency or to reduce intestinal peristalsis and stool frequency. These pharmacologic agents range from mild coating agents or bulk-forming agents to the more widely used antidiarrheal agents (Table 9-2). Of the antidiarrheal agents, loperamide is frequently the drug of choice because of its direct action on the intestinal wall.[43] Loperamide has also been shown to increase the tone of the anorectal smooth muscle, thereby improving continence.

For the patient with diarrhea and incontinence resulting from inflammatory bowel disease, antidiarrheal agents may be used for symptom control in addition to drug therapy for the underlying inflammatory process. Diphenoxylate with atropine (Lomotil) and loperamide (Imodium) are usually effective in con-

Table 9-2 Medications for management of diarrhea

Medication	Action	Side effects	Comments and contraindications
ANTIDIARRHEAL AGENTS			
Cholinergic blockers Atropine sulfate Isopropamide iodide Darbid; Combid Belladonna	Act locally on gut to inhibit intestinal secretions and motility Antispasmodic	Dry mouth; blurred vision; dizziness; headache; dry, flushed skin; drowsiness; tinnitus; vertigo; changes in affect and behavior; vitamin B deficiency	Glaucoma; unstable cardiovascular status; paralytic ileus; chronic lung disease; asthma; pyloric stenosis; liver damage; pregnancy; renal insufficiency; convulsive disorders Administer 30 to 60 min before meal
Opium derivatives Paregoric (tincture of opium) Parapectolin; Diabismul Codeine	Act on smooth muscle of large bowel to increase tone and decrease motility	Addiction Sodium and potassium loss	Dilute in 3 oz of water to ensure absorption in stomach Schedule III drug
Diphenoxylate hydrochloride Lomotil	Act on smooth muscle to inhibit motility and propulsion	Nausea; vomiting; sedation; paralytic ileus; headache	Electrolyte imbalance; liver disease; glaucoma
Loperamide Imodium	Act on smooth and circular muscles to decrease peristalsis and transit time	Nausea; vomiting; skin rash; dry mouth; drowsiness; bloating; gastrointestinal distress	
ABSORPTION AGENTS			
Activated charcoal Charcodote; Darco G-60	Absorb water to firm stool	No adverse effects reported	

Drug	Action	Side Effects/Interactions	Comments
Kaolin and pectin Kaopectate; Pectokay	Protectant and demulcent		Do not administer to patient with pseudomembranous colitis Administer 2 to 3 hr before drugs taken by mouth
Attapulgite Claysorb; Quintess			Useful in cases of traveler's diarrhea
Bismuth subsalicylate Pepto-Bismol	Coating and astringent effects	May decrease effect of anticoagulants Interferes with abdominal radiographs; darkens stool	
BULK-FORMING AGENTS			
Psyllium hydrophilic Mucilloid Konsyl; Effersyllium; Modance Bulk; Metamucil	Absorbs fluid and forms stool bulk	Obstruction with inadequate fluid intake May reduce plasma cholesterol with chronic use; bloating; abdominal distress	Effect within 12 to 24 hours May reduce appetite
ASTRINGENT AND COATING AGENTS			
Aluminum hydroxide Alucal; Amphojel; Nutrajel	Produces barrier between intestinal contents and intestinal wall	Constipation; nausea and vomiting; phosphate deficiency with prolonged use	Do not use with low-sodium diets, tetracycline, or anticoagulants
Bismuth subsalicylate Pepto-Bismol		May decrease effect of anticoagulants; interferes with abdominal radiographs; darkens stool	Useful in cases of traveler's diarrhea
OTHER			
Lactobacillus Lactinex; Moredophilus	Normalizes bowel flora		Used in cases of diarrhea caused by antibiotics. Do not use in patients with high fever; do not use in infants and children under 3 years of age

trolling diarrhea; paregoric and kaolin and pectin (Kaopectate) may also be effective, although they may not be as well tolerated as the former. Caution must be used when combining antidiarrheal agents and anticholinergic drugs in these patients because of the risk of ileus.[43,46]

Fluid and electrolyte replacement. Acute episodes of diarrhea may also place the individual at risk for fluid volume deficit. Nursing intervention must include thorough assessment of fluid-electrolyte balance and measures to prevent or correct deficits. If oral fluids are tolerated, electrolyte solutions such as the electrolyte drinks developed for athletes and ostomy patients may be used to replace losses. A recipe for a homemade electrolyte solution is given in the box below. If oral intake is not tolerated, intravenous replacement may be necessary. Acute diarrhea can be of particular risk to infants and children and must be managed aggressively.

Stool containment. Nursing management of acute diarrhea may include measures to contain and quantify stool until the underlying problem can be corrected. Effective containment measures provide skin protection, improve patient comfort, reduce nursing time, and provide an accurate measurement of fluid losses. External collection devices or internal drainage systems may be used for containment.

EXTERNAL COLLECTION DEVICES

External collection devices designed for the patient with fecal incontinence are available. These devices provide a drainable pouch attached to a synthetic, adhesive skin barrier that is constructed to conform to the perianal area and buttocks. External devices are most effective when applied to clean, dry skin that is free of skin breakdown. If skin breakdown is present, it must be treated (for example, with a skin barrier powder) before the pouch is applied to the area. Guidelines for application of perianal fecal incontinence collectors include

---

HOMEMADE ELECTROLYTE SOLUTION

1 tbsp salt
1 tbsp baking soda
1 tbsp corn syrup
1 can (6 oz) frozen orange juice concentrate

Add water to make one quart of liquid.

Replace fluid volume lost through diarrhea with equivalent volume of solution. If unable to estimate volume of fluid loss, replace with 8 oz of solution for every bowel movement.

the following: perianal hair should be removed, skin barrier paste may be used in the gluteal folds, contact skin adhesive may be used, and a two-person application procedure may be used. (One person supports the patient's buttocks and the second person applies the pouch.)[41,52,54] These devices adhere to the skin for an average of 24 hours or more (Fig. 9-2).

INTERNAL DRAINAGE SYSTEMS

Internal drainage systems are sometimes used when external devices are not feasible because of extensive skin breakdown or lack of adherence.[7] Internal drainage systems involve the use of a large-bore catheter (for example, a French size 30 catheter) that is connected to a bedside drainage bag. Although these systems are used effectively in some settings, many practitioners are concerned that there are no data to support the safety of internal devices. Therefore these systems should be used only on a short-term basis, and strict guidelines for their use should be followed to minimize risk. The use of internal drainage systems is contraindicated in cases of rectal disease, for the immunocompromised patient, and for patients with neutropenia. Guidelines for use vary; some practitioners recommend no inflation or minimal inflation of the catheter balloon, whereas others recommend full inflation with the balloon positioned with light tension just above the anorectal junction. Balloon inflation carries the risk of bowel wall necrosis that results from compression of the microvasculature; if the balloon is inflated, guidelines for frequent deflation to restore blood flow must be strictly followed.

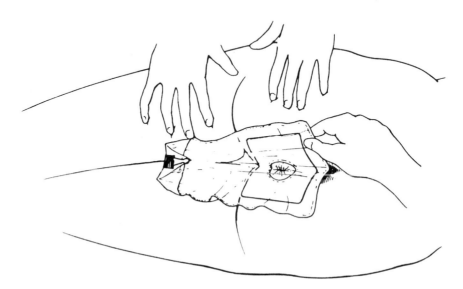

Fig. 9-2   External fecal incontinence collector. (From Vulhop L, Sommers M, and Wolverton C: J Enterost Ther 11:59, 1984.)

A variety of containment products such as incontinence pants is also available for the patient who has severe diarrhea that cannot be managed with external collection devices. The problems of contact dermatitis and odor may limit the use of incontinence pants.

Prevention and management of skin breakdown. Prevention and management of skin breakdown is a major concern in the care of the patient with diarrhea and fecal incontinence.

ROUTINE CARE

Routine skin care should include gentle cleansing of the perianal area after each bowel movement or incontinent episode. Tepid water, pH-balanced soaps, commercial formulas designed for incontinence care, or mineral oil may be used for cleansing. If soaps are used, the skin should be rinsed thoroughly. Manufacturers' instructions for the use of commercial cleansers must be followed, since some products necessitate rinsing and some do not.

After cleansing, intact skin can be protected with a moisture barrier product. The practitioner may choose to coat the skin with a sealant (copolymer film product) and then cover the sealant with a moisture barrier product to provide additional protection. Moisture barrier products are available in both cream and ointment forms; most products contain a petrolatum base and variable other ingredients (for example, lubricants, deodorants, or antibacterial agents). The decision to use a particular brand should be based on available clinical data and on the effectiveness, convenience, availability, and cost of the product.

MANAGEMENT OF DENUDED SKIN

There are several ways to manage denuded skin surfaces caused by contact with liquid stool. One approach is to apply a skin barrier powder to the denuded area; the powder can be used alone, or a moisture barrier product can be applied over the powder. Another approach is to formulate a paste by mixing a skin barrier powder with a moisture barrier product; the paste is used to coat the moist surfaces. (Some practitioners find it helpful to apply the skin barrier powder directly to the moist area to "dry it up" and then apply the paste over the powder.) Recently, premixed ointments and pastes have been introduced by several manufacturers. In some settings, hydrocolloid wafer dressings have been used effectively to manage denuded areas.

MANAGEMENT OF FUNGAL RASH

Patients with fecal incontinence are also at risk for fungal infections (caused by *Candida albicans*), as a result of continual moisture in the perianal area. The risk is increased in patients with diabetes and patients receiving antibiotics or immunosuppressive therapy. Fungal infections typically appear as a maculopapular rash with distinct satellite lesions. An antifungal powder such as nystatin may be dusted onto the area. A sealant or moisture barrier cream may be applied over the powder if needed. Ointments and creams containing antifungal agents have been used, but they appear to lengthen the time required for healing because of the retention of moisture at the skin surface.[34] A broad-spectrum antifungal medication such as imidazole (clotrimazole, miconazole) may be indicated for nonresponsive fungal skin infections, since the infection may be caused by a fungal organism that does not respond to nystatin.[34]

Odor control. A final concern related to diarrhea and incontinence is odor management. If a perianal pouch is used, pouch deodorants are a option. For other patients, deodorizing skin cleansers and effective room-deodorizing sprays may be used to eliminate offensive odors.

Constipation

Pathophysiology. Constipation is another aspect of altered stool consistency that may contribute to fecal incontinence. As discussed earlier in this chapter, unrelieved constipation or impaction may first appear to be diarrhea and fecal incontinence. When an impaction is present, watery stool seeps around the obstructing fecal mass. If antidiarrheal agents are then given, cycles of constipation, impaction, and diarrhea may develop. Chronic constipation may also cause loss of normal rectal tone; as a result the individual no longer senses rectal fullness and does not voluntarily contract the external sphincter, and stool leakage occurs.

Constipation may be caused by inadequate intake of fluids and dietary bulk that results in small, hard, dry stools or by reduced peristaltic activity as a result of aging, inactivity, the abuse of laxatives or enemas or both, metabolic disease, or narcotics.[1,5,13,27,37] Poor bowel hygiene (prolonged failure to defecate) is also a causative factor for chronic constipation and related incontinence.[5,27]

Management. For the person with chronic constipation, restoration of normal stool consistency is the first step in treatment. Achievement of soft, bulky stool depends on adequate intake of fiber and fluids. Fiber can be supplied by dietary modifications, bran or bran mixtures, or bulk agents.[12,21] Bran and bran mixtures have been reported to be effective in restoring normal stool consistency and regularity of defecation. The usual initial dosage of bran is 1 to 2 tbsp taken one or two times a day, with subsequent doses titrated based on individual response. Increased stool frequency and flatus may occur during the first 2 to 3 weeks of bran therapy; regularity is usually established within 1 month.

Bulk-forming agents such as psyllium seed derivatives also provide dietary fiber. These products work by absorbing fluid in the bowel and must be used in combination with adequate fluid intake.

Combination agents that contain stool softeners and peristaltic stimulants may also be prescribed for patients with constipation. Although these combination agents are effective when used properly, in most situations the addition of fiber, along with adequate fluid intake, increased activity, and avoidance of constipating medications, is enough to promote the desired soft, bulky stool.[27]

Table 9-3   Medications for the management of constipation

Medication	Action	Side effects	Comments and contraindications
BULK-FORMING AGENTS			
Karaya Methylcellulose Cologel; Hydrolose Psyllium Metamucil; Konsyl; Modance Bulk; Effersyllium	Absorbs water in gastrointestinal tract to soften stool and increase stool size	May increase flatus for 1 to 2 weeks; abdominal cramping	May be unpalatable; bolus formation with inadequate fluid intake
FECAL SOFTENERS AND LUBRICANTS			
Mineral oil	Emulsifies fats; lubricates and softens stool	May affect gastrointestinal absorption; may affect absorption of fat-soluble vitamins (A, D, E, and K)	Instruct patients to sit up for several hours after ingestion to prevent lipid pneumonia; oil may seep from rectum
Dioctyl sodium sulfosuccinate Surfak Dioctyl calcium sulfosuccinate Colace; DDS Glycerine suppository	Surface-active agent that allows water to penetrate stool		Works well in combination with bisacodyl suppository for patients with sensory and motor deficits Place suppository against rectal wall

	Action	Adverse effects	Comments
SALINE CATHARTICS Magnesium hydroxide Magnesium citrate Epsom salts Lactulose	Retains water in small bowel and increases fluid in colon Osmotic catharsis	Excessive absorption of medications in bowel; may be difficult to return bowel function to normal if used regularly	Unpleasant effects; effective in patients receiving chemotherapy or patients with narcotic-induced constipation, when other interventions are not effective

STIMULANT CATHARTICS
Bisacodyl
  Dulcolax; Bisco-Lax
Senna
Cascara
  Cas-evac; Bileo-Secrin
	Stimulates parasympathetic reflexes to produce peristalsis	Irritating to rectum; electrolyte imbalance; myenteric plexus degeneration with prolonged use	Habit-forming; effective for upper motor neuron lesions; must not be used with alkaline agents (antacids)

Castor oil		Emulsified castor oil turns alkaline urine pink.	
OTHER Carbon dioxide evacuant	Releases carbon dioxide into rectum to stimulate peristalsis	May cause autonomic dysreflexia	Expensive; may be used during bowel training for patient with loss of anorectal reflex

Table 9-3 includes common substances used in the treatment of constipation and their mechanisms of action.

BOWEL TRAINING
Candidates for Bowel Training

Alterations in sensory awareness or sphincter control may result in incontinence; these patients may be helped by bowel training programs, exercises to tone muscles, biofeedback therapy, or combinations of these programs.[11,22,44,48,57] Individuals with sensory or motor deficits or both who may benefit from bowel training programs include those with spinal cord injury, spina bifida, congenital anorectal defects, and neurologic conditions. Older individuals with sensory or sphincter deficits may also benefit from such programs. Children with encopresis may also benefit from bowel training; these children have prolonged failure to defecate that results in stool retention, constipation, and overflow incontinence.[16,53,55]

Factors That Affect Success

A successful bowel training program is based on assessment of the person's functional ability, cognitive status, motivation, current bowel habits and stool consistency, current and past use of bowel stimulants, and dietary intake. A bowel training program is developed in collaboration with the patient or caregiver; the program is based on assessment data and should offer a practical approach to restoring regular bowel movements and eliminating fecal soiling and incontinence. Regular bowel movements (daily or every other day) can usually be achieved within several weeks for the adult, whereas a period of several months may be required to develop a workable and successful program for children.[11,13] The components of a successful bowel training program are identified in the box on p. 253.

Preliminary Measures. Preliminary measures include elimination of any impacted stool, environmental manipulation to facilitate continence, and active involvement of the patient or caregiver. The establishment of regular, soft, bulky stools is also addressed, as discussed earlier in this chapter.

Establishment of Voluntary Control. Voluntary control of defecation is established if possible.
Patient with intact sensory and motor function. The patient with intact sensory and motor pathways learns to use known stimuli to initiate defecation on a regular basis, and the patient is taught and encouraged to respond to the sensation of rectal fullness. For the individual with diminished sensory awareness, sensory retraining may be beneficial.[56]

BOWEL TRAINING PROGRAM

1. Obtain bowel history and establish a schedule for the bowel training program that is normal and comfortable for the patient and conforms to his or her lifestyle.
2. Ensure adequate fiber and fluid intake. (Normalize stool consistency.)
   Fiber
      Add high-fiber foods to diet (dried fruit, dried beans, vegetables, and wheat products).
      Suggest adding 1 to 3 tbsp bran or Metamucil to diet one or two times a day. (Titrate dosage based on response.)
   Fluid
      Two to 3 liters daily (unless contraindicated)
      Four ounces of prune, fig, or pear juice (or a warm fluid) may be given daily as a stimulus (for example, 30 minutes to 1 hour before the established time for defecation).
3. Encourage exercise program.
   Pelvic tilt, modified sit-ups for abdominal strength
   Walking for general muscle tone and cardiovascular system
   More vigorous program if appropriate
4. Establish a regular time for the bowel movement.
   Established time depends on patient's schedule.

Best times are 20 to 40 minutes after regularly scheduled meals, when gastrocolic reflex is active.
Attempts at evacuation should be made daily within 15 minutes of the established time and whenever the patient senses rectal distention.
Instruct patient in normal posture for defecation. (The patient normally sits on the toilet or bedside commode; for the patient who is unable to get out of bed, the left side-lying position is best.)
Instruct the patient to contract the abdominal muscles and "bear down."
Have patient lean forward to increase the intra-abdominal pressure by use of compression against the thighs.
Stimulate anorectal reflex and rectal emptying if necessary.
   Insert a rectal suppository or mini-enema into the rectum 15 to 30 minutes before the scheduled bowel movement, placing the suppository against the bowel wall, or
   Insert a gloved, lubricated finger into the anal canal and gently dilate the anal sphincter.

Patient with sensory or motor deficit. If a patient has a sensory deficit or a loss of external sphincter function (for example, the patient with spinal cord injury or spina bifida), rectal evacuation is routinely stimulated at a time that is convenient for that individual or caregiver. For the individual who works or attends school, evening hours are usually preferable.

A commonly used approach for initiating rectal evacuation is digital stimulation.[39] A gloved, lubricated finger is inserted into the anal canal, and a circular motion is used (for 30 seconds to 2 minutes) until the sphincter relaxes. If results do not occur within 20 minutes after this procedure, digital stimulation may be repeated.[13] In some rehabilitation centers, digital stimulation is continued without interruption until rectal evacuation occurs or for a maximum period of 20 minutes.

Bisacodyl or glycerine suppositories may also be used to stimulate evacuation. Common complaints with this option are delayed response and inconsistent or incomplete rectal evacuation or both. To be effective the suppository must be inserted against the rectal wall, not into the fecal mass.[50]

Docusate and glycerine are also available as a liquid, single-dose, 4 ml minienema, which eliminates the delay associated with the need to wait for a solid suppository to melt; limited studies of the mini-enema have shown improved rectal evacuation and faster response time.[9]

Other measures that promote rectal evacuation include the following:[11,19,37]

1. Timing evacuation to coincide with the gastrocolic stimulus (just after a meal, when the gastrocolic reflex is active)
2. Placing the individual in a squat position to achieve the proper angle between the rectum and the anal canal
3. Instructing the patient to contract the abdominal muscles to increase intra-abdominal pressures

Once the regular defecation response has been established, the use of suppositories and digital stimulation may be eliminated for some patients; defecation can be achieved with the gastrocolic reflex and contraction of the abdominal muscles.

Use of enemas for bowel training is generally contraindicated because of the potential to create bowel dependency. In selected individuals the use of enemas may help maintain regular bowel function and prevent skin breakdown; the use of enemas is most appropriate for the older patient in whom rehabilitation is not feasible and who does not respond well to lesser stimuli (such as suppositories). In this situation it may be helpful to administer the enema with a cone tip (such as the tip used for colostomy irrigations) or with the nipple of a baby bottle fitted around the tip of the catheter to prevent backflow.

In any bowel program, consistency is crucial to success. Adequate follow-up, modifications as necessary, and ongoing support increase the potential for a successful outcome.

SENSORY REEDUCATION

When a patient has diminished sensory awareness or reduced sphincter control, sensory reeducation or sphincter retraining may be beneficial. These therapies are usually best provided in an anorectal physiology clinic. These clinics are equipped to provide evaluation of the person with incontinence and to support biofeedback therapy. Standard evaluation includes assessment of internal and external sphincter function and evaluation of the anorectal sensory mechanisms.[56] These evaluation procedures are discussed in detail in Chapter 8.

The anorectal sensory mechanisms allow for discrimination of the character of the enteric contents (gas, liquid, or solid stool) and detection of the need to pass that content. A deficit in sensory mechanisms may result in incontinence in two ways. (1) If the presence of rectal distention cannot be sensed and the external sphincter is not contracted, gas and stool may escape. (2) If rectal distention is not recognized and the person does not voluntarily defecate, solid stool may accumulate in the rectum and lead to constipation and overflow incontinence. The latter is often the case in young children who have ignored the "call to stool" for long periods.

If a sensory deficit is evident on anorectal manometry, the individual must be retrained to recognize rectal distention.[56] This retraining can be accomplished by inserting a catheter with a balloon tip into the person's rectum and initially inflating the balloon to the level of the first sensation of pressure. The degree of inflation is progressively reduced until the sensation is within normal limits (15 to 30 cc).

SPHINCTER RETRAINING
Indications

If a person is unable to voluntarily contract the external sphincter when the rectal vault fills, stool leakage may occur. Sphincter retraining may be beneficial for these patients when the following criteria are met: (1) A weak but contractable external sphincter muscle is present and (2) Anatomic defects are minimal or absent. Sphincter retraining may not be effective when there are large amounts of scar tissue (from episiotomy or surgical procedure) or severe congenital defects. The success of sphincter retraining depends on the patient's motivation and ability to comprehend and follow instructions. Sphincter retraining has been successful in the following specific situations*:

1. Anorectal surgery: hemorrhoidectomy, imperforate anus repair, subtotal proctectomy, rectal prolapse repair, and ileoanal anastomosis
2. Medical conditions: inflammatory bowel disease of the rectum, diabetes, radiation enteritis, or scleroderma

*References 14, 17, 44, 48, 58, and 59.

3. Neurologic deficits: cerebrovascular accidents, Hirschsprung's disease, laminectomy, or myelomeningocele
4. Psychosomatic conditions: irritable bowel syndrome or encopresis

Procedures

Pelvic Floor Exercises. Sphincter retraining includes pelvic floor exercises with or without biofeedback therapy. Repeated tightening of the pelvic floor muscle results in increased muscle tone and increased ability to prevent stool leakage. The benefits of these exercises were first reported by Arnold Kegel in 1948 and are commonly known as Kegel exercises.[29]

The first step in a pelvic floor or Kegel exercise program is to have the person identify the correct muscle by squeezing as tightly as possible around a finger placed in the anal canal or vagina. Another method for isolating the correct muscle is to instruct the individual to stop urine flow in midstream and concentrate on the muscle used. The identified muscle is held in a squeeze for a count of 10 and then relaxed for a count of 10. The exercise should be performed 20 to 25 times, three times a day.

Kegel exercises can be performed while standing, sitting, or lying down. Consistent daily exercise is the key to increasing muscle tone. The exercises should be incorporated into the patient's daily life-style to provide maximum benefit. When these exercises have been taught and practiced properly, they have proved effective in reducing incontinence.[29,30] A problem with the use of exercise programs alone is that some people have difficulty in identifying the correct muscle group and performing the exercise properly. Exercise programs that incorporate biofeedback are now available and appear to increase the success rate of sphincter retraining.

Biofeedback Therapy. Biofeedback therapy is an easy and safe method of treatment for certain individuals with incontinence.[44,57,60] Broadly defined, biofeedback therapy is the use of instrumentation to mirror psychophysiologic processes that the individual is not normally aware of and that may be controlled voluntarily. The mechanism by which biofeedback works is not understood; however, studies of patients who have used biofeedback therapy have documented an increase in the patients' sense of control and a decrease in feelings of helplessness and anxiety.[50]

Currently two methods of biofeedback therapy for the treatment of fecal incontinence are popular. Cerulli[14] and Whitehead[59] described a manometric device with three balloons that provides feedback on a recording apparatus (see Fig. 8-17, p. 225). MacLeod[36] used a rectal plug that provided feedback from an electromyogram (EMG) or a computer monitor (Fig. 9-3). With either approach a sensing device is inserted into the rectum and baseline resting and squeeze pressure readings are recorded. The individual is then taught how to

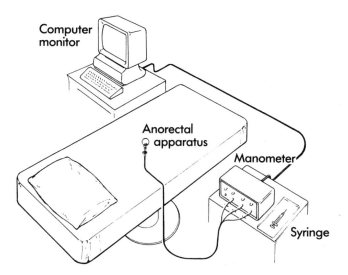

Fig. 9-3   Rectal plug device for EMG feedback.

squeeze the external sphincter muscle around the balloon or plug. Changes in the pressures are visualized on a strip recording or a video monitor so that the person receives immediate feedback; this reinforces the squeeze sensation. (With some systems the patient receives auditory feedback.) In some settings an EMG reading is also taken of the abdominal muscles and puborectalis muscle; this reading demonstrates any inappropriate contractions of the abdominal muscles and provides the person with visual correlation between contractions of the external sphincter and the puborectalis. Sessions last from 30 minutes to 2 hours. Training is completed in an average of three sessions. Sensory training during biofeedback therapy is also achievable with each of these methods.

Controversy exists as to the better method of retraining the pelvic floor musculature, that is, exercises alone versus exercises with biofeedback therapy. Whitehead[58] showed that biofeedback therapy did result in greater improvement in continence than did the use of pelvic floor exercises alone. Most current programs use the biofeedback technique weekly in the clinic setting, and patients supplement this biofeedback therapy by doing pelvic floor exercises at home.

Success of the biofeedback program can be measured both objectively and subjectively. Although manometric studies performed after biofeedback therapy do not always show a significant improvement in sphincter tone, several authors have reported a success rate of 70% to 90% as described by their patients.[36,44,58]

Individuals consider biofeedback therapy successful if the quality of their lives is improved.

MANAGEMENT OF REDUCED RECTAL CAPACITY AND COMPLIANCE

Fecal incontinence and frequency may also be present when rectal capacity or compliance or both decrease. In such cases a given volume of stool within the rectum produces high pressures that exceed the anal sphincter pressures and result in urgency and incontinence. The initial goal of management should be to correct the underlying disease (for example, inflammatory conditions that affect the rectum). For some patients a daily program of progressively larger retention enemas is effective in increasing rectal compliance and capacity.[60] For severe, irreversible damage to the rectum (for example, radiation proctitis) that results in constant tenesmus and incontinence, fecal diversion may be considered.

SURGICAL MANAGEMENT

Patients with incontinence that has not improved during a well-regimented, well-documented conservative treatment plan or patients with incontinence that is not amenable to conservative therapy may be candidates for surgical

---

INDICATIONS FOR SURGICAL INTERVENTION IN MANAGEMENT OF FECAL INCONTINENCE

TRAUMATIC
Obstetric (childbirth)
Surgical injury
Accidental injuries (blunt or penetrating)

IDIOPATHIC
Associated with aging
Associated with procidentia

NEUROGENIC
Accidental injuries
Central nervous system or spinal cord injuries

CONGENITAL
Imperforate anus
Spina bifida
Hirschsprung's disease

MEDICAL
Radiation enteritis
Inflammatory bowel disease

intervention.[16] The most common indications for surgery are listed in the box on p. 258.

Before surgery is considered,[23] a thorough history and physical (including studies of anorectal physiology) should be performed and the underlying pathophysiology of the incontinence should be established. The surgical procedure of choice depends on the specific dysfunction.

Surgical intervention should be designed to correct the abnormal continence mechanism. The availability of many procedures suggests that no single procedure is best for all individuals and that these procedures are not easy to perform, nor are they free of complications.

Sphincter Repair

For patients who have a deficient external sphincter with no neurologic damage, a direct anal sphincter repair can be performed. Sphincter repair is accomplished by the apposition or the overlapping of the muscle.[18] With either procedure the ends of the external sphincter muscle are identified and lifted. The ends are sewn end to end (apposition) or overlapped. The overlap procedure offers a margin of security that allows for some muscle retraction without complete disruption of the repair (Fig. 9-4).

When incontinence caused by aging or procidentia occurs, the muscles are usually intact but poorly functioning with or without a straight anorectal angle. A Parks postanal repair is usually the surgery of choice in this situation. The procedure involves tacking the levator ani muscles posteriorly in an attempt

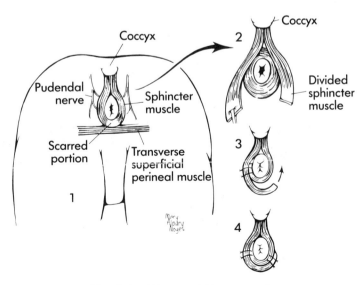

Fig. 9-4   Direct sphincter repair.

to improve continence by making the anal rectal angle more acute and lengthening the anal canal (Fig. 9-5).[40]

The nurse cares for these patients postoperatively by focusing on pain management and bowel function. Most patients have a great deal of pain after a sphincter repair procedure. Currently this pain is managed by a continuous epidural pain block for the first 2 to 3 days after surgery. When the epidural pain block is used, the patient's respiratory rate and level of sedation must be monitored.

As a result of analgesics, decreased activity, alteration in diet, and perineal edema, constipation is often a problem after surgery. To restore proper bowel function, bulk agents and daily tap water enemas may be necessary initially.[40] It is sometimes difficult to distinguish the anal canal opening from the surgical wound. The anal canal opening is best identified by locating the coccyx and inserting the enema tip just anterior to it. The wound can then be located on the anterior aspect of the anal opening.

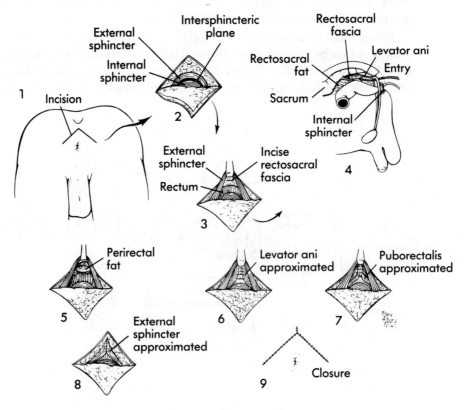

Fig. 9-5   Parks postanal repair.

Although anal sphincter repair is a minor procedure, the postoperative period is often stressful because of the difficulty in dealing with the pain and returning bowel function to normal.

Gracilis Muscle Transfer

When neurogenic incontinence occurs because of the loss of innervation to the sphincter muscle, the gracilis muscle transfer procedure may be performed.[18] The gracilis muscle, taken from the inner aspect of the thigh, is brought around to encircle the anus (Fig. 9-6). Because this encirclement is of living tissue, the muscle can stretch and contract during defecation. Leguit reported on 10 patients with a follow-up period of 6 months to 17 years: 90% of the patients were continent for formed stool; one patient reported no improvement.[32]

Artificial Sphincter

Christenson[15] and Wong[61] have recently reported the use of a Silastic artificial bowel sphincter for patients who are not candidates for or who have failed traditional surgical repair. The individual controls defecation by deflating a cuff mechanism placed around the external sphincter muscle. The cuff automatically reinflates over a period of 10 minutes to provide continence. Although

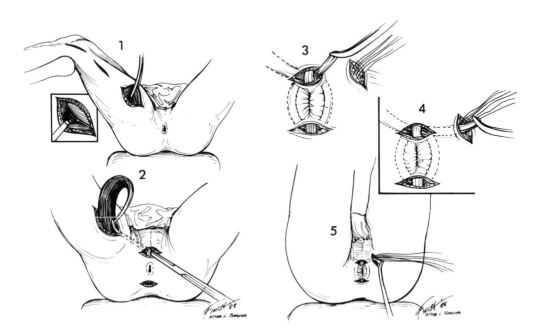

Fig. 9-6　Gracilis muscle transfer.

the series studied in each case is small, the early results are promising. This procedure appears to be an exciting new alternative for the surgical management of fecal incontinence.

Bowel Resection

When a disease process (for example, ulcerative colitis or radiation enteritis) contributes to diarrhea and fecal incontinence, procedures such as the ileoanal reservoir are options for management. This approach involves elimination of the disease process rather than alteration of the sphincter mechanism.

Fecal Diversion

Fecal diversion is now playing less of a role in the management of fecal incontinence than it did in the past, although it is still an option for those who have a disease not amenable to alternative therapies.

SUMMARY

The management of fecal incontinence can be approached in many ways. For all individuals a thorough assessment of the problem and correction of identified causes is the initial focus. When conservative measures fail, more aggressive interventions, ranging from sphincter retraining to medications or surgery or both may be necessary. Finally, containment of the stool and odor and protection of the skin must be provided to restore the comfort and dignity of the person with intractable fecal incontinence.

SELF-EVALUATION

QUESTIONS

1. Identify environmental modifications that facilitate toileting and continence for the ambulatory person.
2. Identify at least two causes of chronic diarrhea.
3. Identify data to be recorded in a diet and stool history form.
4. Explain the purpose and procedure for an elimination diet.
5. Which of the following is caused by a common enzyme deficiency?
   a. Lactose intolerance
   b. Celiac disease
   c. Caffeine sensitivity
   d. Alcohol-related diarrhea
6. Explain why elemental diets may be beneficial to the patient with severe malabsorption and diarrhea.
7. List at least two common causes of acute diarrhea.
8. Explain why enteral feedings may cause diarrhea, and identify appropriate nursing interventions.
9. Explain why bulk-forming laxatives may be used for the patient with diarrhea, as well as for the patient with constipation.
10. Which of the following is the drug of choice for diarrhea?
    a. Diphenoxylate (Lomotil)
    b. Loperamide (Imodium)
    c. Kaolin and pectin compounds (Kaopectate)
    d. Codeine
11. Identify one safe method for containment and quantification of liquid stool.
12. Describe potential complications of internal fecal drainage systems and implications for nursing care.
13. Identify the principles of skin care for the patient with fecal incontinence.
14. Describe two methods for management of denuded skin.
15. Identify factors that may cause or contribute to constipation.
16. Identify three methods of providing adequate intake of fiber.
17. Which of the following patients is *not* a candidate for a bowel training program?
    a. Child with encopresis
    b. Adult with sensory deficits and constipation
    c. Adult with diarrhea secondary to inflammatory bowel disease
    d. Teenager with incontinence caused by spinal cord injury
18. Jesse Thompson is an 8-year-old boy with spina bifida who has been referred for bowel training. Currently his bowel pattern is one of cycles of constipation, impaction, and diarrhea; he does not sense rectal fullness and can-

not control his external sphincter. Which of the following measures should *not* be included in a bowel training program for Jesse?

a. Establishment of regular schedule (for example, every other day after supper) for bowel program

b. Initial disimpaction as necessary

c. Provision for increased fiber and fluids

d. Instruction to respond promptly to feelings of rectal distention (that is, tell Jesse to go to the bathroom and contract his abdominal muscles to help push stool out).

19. Which of the following stimulants should *not* be used routinely in bowel training programs?

a. Digital stimulation

b. Suppositories

c. Enemas

d. Mini-enemas

20. Sensory reeducation is designed to restore:

a. Discrimination of gas, liquid, and solid

b. Internal sphincter control

c. Awareness of rectal distention

d. External sphincter control

21. Identify candidates for sphincter retraining programs, including indications and factors that affect the success of the retraining programs.

22. Explain why biofeedback therapy may be beneficial in a sphincter retraining program.

23. Identify treatment options for the patient with reduced rectal capacity and compliance.

24. The patient with neurogenic impairment of sphincter function is most likely to benefit from:

a. Direct sphincter repair

b. Parks postanal repair

c. Anorectal transplant

d. Gracilis muscle transfer

SELF-EVALUATION

ANSWERS

1. Easily accessible and clearly marked toilet facilities
   Adequate lighting
   Toilet facilities accessible to persons who use walkers
   Handrails or grab bars in hallways and bathrooms
   Toilets and commodes at appropriate height for independent entry and exit
   Clothing that facilitates toileting

2. **a.** Dietary intolerance
   b. Malabsorption syndromes
   c. Intestinal disorders that cause excessive motility

3. **a.** Types and amounts of foods and fluids ingested, including time of intake
   b. Types and amounts of fecal output, including time of defecation

4. Purpose: Identify and eliminate foods that are poorly tolerated
   Procedure: Begin by eliminating foods that commonly cause symptoms of intolerance and foods identified as suspect by diet and stool history. Once symptoms are controlled, reintroduce foods one at a time; isolate and restrict those that exacerbate symptoms.

5. **a.** Lactose intolerance

6. Elemental diets provide nutrients in simplified, ready-to-absorb form; digestion is unnecessary, so absorption in the small bowel is maximized.

7. **a.** Unrecognized impaction
   b. Gastroenteritis
   c. Intestinal candidiasis
   d. Enteral feedings in the malnourished patient

8. Enteral feedings may cause diarrhea because the formula is hypertonic; more commonly diarrhea is caused by an underlying malnutrition with associated bowel wall edema or atrophy of the villi or both, which results in malabsorption.
   Nursing interventions include selection of an isotonic formula; initiation of feeding at a slow rate (approximately 50 ml/hr); measures to control diarrhea as necessary (for example, the use of formula with fiber; the use of antidiarrheal medications).

9. Bulk-forming agents act by absorbing fluid in the bowel. For the patient with diarrhea this absorption acts as a stool thickener; for the patient with constipation it softens and adds bulk to the stool. Bulk-forming agents tend to normalize stool consistency.

10. **b.** Loperamide (Imodium)

11. Use of a fecal incontinence collector

12. Potential complications include tissue necrosis secondary to prolonged inflation of the catheter balloon and sphincter damage caused by prolonged use of indwelling rectal catheter.

Nursing implications include the following:

Use of external collection devices instead of internal drainage systems whenever possible

Restriction of the use of internal drainage systems to short-term use, and use only with patients with no rectal disease or disorder who are not neutropenic or immunosuppressed

No inflation or minimal inflation of the catheter balloon: if the catheter balloon is inflated, it must be deflated at frequent intervals to prevent necrosis

13. **a.** Gentle cleansing after each incontinent episode (with water, pH-balanced soap, or commercial cleanser)
   b. Use of skin sealants or moisture barrier products (creams and ointments) or both to protect intact skin.

14. **a.** Skin barrier powder is applied to the denuded area; moisture barrier product is applied over the powder.
   b. Hydrocolloid wafer dressing is applied to the denuded area.
   c. Paste made of skin barrier powder and moisture barrier product is applied to the denuded surface. (Skin barrier powder may be applied to the denuded surface before it is coated with paste.)

15. **a.** Inadequate intake of dietary fluids and bulk, which results in small, hard, dry stools
   b. Inactivity, aging, abuse of laxatives or enemas or both, metabolic disease, and use of narcotics, which cause reduced peristalsis
   c. Prolonged failure to defecate

16. **a.** Dietary modifications
   b. Daily consumption of bran or bran mixture
   c. Use of bulk-forming laxatives

17. **c.** Adult with diarrhea secondary to inflammatory bowel disease

18. **d.** Instruction to respond promptly to feelings of rectal distention

19. **c.** Enemas

20. **c.** Awareness of rectal distention

21. Patients with deficient external sphincter control who have a weak but contractable sphincter muscle, have minimal or absent, anatomic defects are able to follow directions, and are motivated.

22. In sphincter retraining programs, patients often have difficulty with consistent isolation of the correct muscle; biofeedback therapy includes the use of sensors connected to recording devices that display the patient's responses; this display provides the patient with immediate visual feedback during contraction of the desired muscle.

23. **a.** Treatment of underlying disease process
   b. Use of progressively larger retention enemas
   c. Fecal diversion

24. **d.** Gracilis muscle transfer

REFERENCES

1. Alterescu V: Theoretical foundations for an approach to fecal incontinence, J Enterost Ther 13:44, 1986.
2. Alun-Jones V et al: Crohn's disease: maintenance of remission by diet, Lancet 1:177, 1985.
3. American Dietetic Association: Manual of clinical dietetics, Chicago, 1988, The Association.
4. Anderson J et al: Candidiasis hypersensitivity syndrome, J Allergy Clin Immunol 78:271, 1986.
5. Basch A: Changes in elimination, Semin Oncol Nurs 3:4, 1987.
6. Bayliss T: Nutritional therapy of IBD, Endoscopy Rev 4:4, 1987.
7. Birdsall C: Would you put a Foley in the rectum? Am J Nurs 9:1050DD, 1986.
8. Bralow S and Marks G: Radiation injury to the gut. In Bockus E, ed: Gastroenterology, Philadelphia, 1985, WB Saunders Co.
9. Brier L and Benedict A: Eliminating suppositories in bowel training, Am J Nurs 86:522, 1986.
10. Brinson R and Kotts B: Hypoalbuminemia as an indicator of diarrheal incidence in critically ill patients, Crit Care Med 15:506, 1987.
11. Brunner L: Manual of nursing practice, ed 4, Philadelphia, 1986, JB Lippincott Co.
12. Burkitt DP, Walker ARP, and Painter, NS: Effect of dietary fiber on stools and transit times and its role in the causation of disease, Lancet 12:1408, 1972.
13. Carlsen C, Griggs W, and King R, eds: Rehabilitation nursing procedures manual, Rockville, MD, 1990, Aspen Publishers, Inc.
14. Cerulli M, Nikoomanesh P, and Schuster M: Progress in biofeedback conditioning for fecal incontinence, Gastroenterology 76:742, 1979.
15. Christenson J and Lorentzen M: Implantation of the artificial sphincter for anal incontinence, Dis Colon Rectum 32:432, 1989.
16. Cohen M et al: Rationale for medical or surgical therapy in anal incontinence, Dis Colon Rectum 29:120, 1986.
17. Coller JA: Clinical applications of anorectal manometry, Gastroenterol Clin North Am 61:17, 1987.
18. Corman MC: Gracilis muscle transposition for anal incontinence: late results, Br J Surg 72[Suppl]:S21, 1985.
19. Corman ML: The management of anal incontinence, Surg Clin North Am 63:177, 1983.
20. Crook W: The yeast connection: a medical breakthrough, ed 2, Jackson, Tenn, 1984, Professional Books, Inc.
21. Davis A et al: Bowel management: a quality assurance approach to upgrading programs, J Gerontol Nurs 12:13, 1989.
22. Dodge J, Bachman C, and Silverman H: Fecal incontinence in the elderly, Postgrad Med 83:258, 1988.
23. Fazio VW: Current therapy in colon and rectal surgery, Philadelphia, 1989, BC Decker, Inc.
24. Frick O et al: A sensible approach to food allergy, Patient Care 19:48, 1985.
25. Gauvreau J et al: Nutritional management of patients with intestinal graft-versus-host disease, J Am Diet Assoc 79:673, 1981.
26. Ginsgerg A: New treatments for inflammatory bowel disease, Endoscopy Rev 9:24, 1987.
27. Gross J: Elimination: functional alterations–bowel. In Johnson B and Gross J, eds: Handbook of oncology nursing, Bethany, Conn, 1985, Fleschner Publishing Co.
28. Harju E: Dietary habits in patients with dumping syndrome–like symptoms after proximal selective vagotomy, J Clin Gastroenterol 8:5, 1986.
29. Kegel A: Progressive resistive exercises in the functional restoration of the perineal muscles, Am J Obstet Gynecol 56:238, 1948.
30. Kegel A: Stress incontinence of women: psychological treatment, J Int Coll Surg 25:484, 1956.
31. Kregs G and Rodtran J: Diarrhea in gastrointestinal disease. In Sleisenger M and Rodtran J, eds: Gastrointestinal disease, ed 3, Philadelphia, 1983, WB Saunders Co.
32. Leguit P, Van Baal JG, and Brummelkamp WH: Gracilis muscle transposition in the treatment of fecal incontinence: long-term followup and evaluation of anal pressure recordings, Dis Colon Rectum 28:1, 1985.
33. Leonard T, Watson R, and Mohs M: The effects of caffeine on various body systems: a review, J Am Diet Assoc 87:8, 1987.

34. Lookingbill D and Marks J: Principles of dermatology, Philadelphia, 1986, WB Saunders Co.

35. Lorenzo C et al: Pectin delays gastric emptying and increases satiety in obese subjects, Gastroenterology 95:1211, 1988.

36. MacLeod J: Management of anal incontinence by biofeedback, Gastroenterology 93:291, 1987.

37. McLane A: Constipation. In Thompson JM et al, eds: Clinical nursing, ed 2, St Louis, 1989, Mosby–Year Book, Inc.

38. McMahon K and Coyne N: Symptom management in patients with AIDS, Semin Oncol Nurs 5:289, 1989.

39. Norton C: Nursing for continence, Beaconsfield, England, 1986, Beaconsfield Publishers Ltd.

40. Parks AG: Anorectal incontinence, Proc R Soc Med 68:681, 1975.

41. Peterson M: Effective fecal collectors, J Enterost Ther 15:259, 1988.

42. Rao SSC, Read NW, and Holdsworth CD: Is the diarrhoea in ulcerative colitis related to impaired colonic salvage of carbohydrate? Gut 28:1090, 1987.

43. Read M et al: Effects of loperamide on anal sphincter function in patients complaining of chronic diarrhea with fecal incontinence and urgency, Dig Dis Sci 27:807, 1982.

44. Riboli EB et al: Biofeedback conditioning for fecal incontinence, Arch Phys Med Rehabil 69:29, 1988.

45. Rombeau R: Enteral and parenteral nutrition in patients with enteric fistulas and short bowel syndrome, Surg Clin North Am 63:551, 1987.

46. Schuman B: Inflammatory bowel disease, Postgrad Med 83:4, 1988.

47. Schwartz D and Darrow K: Hypoalbuminemia-induced diarrhea in the enterally alimented patient, Nutr Support Specialist 306:235, 1988.

48. Schwartz M: Biofeedback: a practitioner's guide, New York, 1987, The Guilford Press.

49. Smith D: Personal correspondence, June 5, 1990.

50. Smith D and Newman D: Nursing manual on incontinence and other related bladder and bowel disorders, Philadelphia, 1988, Golden Horizons, Inc.

51. Strober W: Gluten-sensitive enteropathy: a nonallergic immune hypersensitivity of the gastrointestinal tract, J Allergy Clin Immunol 78:202, 1986.

52. Symposium highlights: physiology, diagnosis, and therapy in GI motility disorders, Dig Dis Week, 1987.

53. Toth L: Alterations in bowel elimination. In Mitchell PH, ed: AANN's neuroscience nursing, East Norwalk, Conn, 1988, Appleton & Lange.

54. Vulhop L, Sommers M, and Wolverton C: Containment of fecal incontinence by the use of a perianal pouch, J Enterost Ther 11:59, 1984.

55. Wald A: Childhood encopresis: candidates identified for biofeedback therapy, Gastroenterology Observer 6:2, 1987.

56. Wald A: Anorectal sensorimotor dysfunction in fecal incontinence and diabetes mellitus, New Engl J Med 310:20, 1984.

57. Whitehead WE, Burgio KL, and Engel BT: Biofeedback treatment of fecal incontinence in geriatric patients, J Am Geriatr Soc 33:320, 1985.

58. Whitehead WE and Schuster MM: Anorectal physiology and pathophysiology, Am J Gastroenterol 82:487, 1987.

59. Whitehead WE et al: Treatment of fecal incontinence in children with spina bifida: comparison of biofeedback and behavior modification, Arch Phys Med Rehabil 76:218, 1986.

60. Wong WD: Personal correspondence, May 15, 1990.

61. Wong WD and Rothenberger DA: Surgical approaches to anal incontinence. In Brock G and Whalen J, eds: Neurobiology of incontinence, New York, 1990, John Wiley & Sons, Inc.

Index

Get The Whole Picture
With
Volumes II and III
Of The
Enterostomal Therapy Nursing Series

VOLUME II
ACUTE AND CHRONIC WOUNDS:
Nursing Management
Ruth Bryant, RN, MS, CETN
February 1992 (0-8016-0896-1)

- Provides a comprehensive discussion of anatomy and physiology of skin and basic skin care.
- Covers wound assessment, the physiology of wound healing, and acute wound management.
- Explains the role of good nutrition in proper wound healing.
- Includes all the latest techniques for managing pressure and vascular ulcers, draining wounds and fistulas, and per-cutaneous tubes.

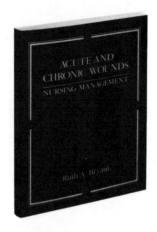

VOLUME III
OSTOMIES AND CONTINENT
DIVERSIONS: Nursing Management
Beverly Hampton, RN, MSN, CETN, ONC
June 1992 (0-8016-2041-4)

- Reviews anatomy and physiology of the GI and GU tracts.
- Explains the indications for surgical construction of urinary and fecal ostomies and continent diversions.
- Equips the nurse to effectively manage and rehabilitate the patient with an ostomy or continent diversion.
- Features a section on oncology con-siderations for practitioners who specialize in cancer care.

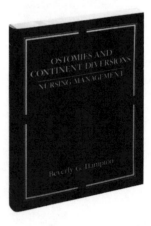

To order ask your bookstore manager or call toll-free 800-426-4545. We look forward to hearing from you soon.

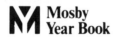
Mosby
Year Book

NMA068

DATE DUE

The Library Store   #47-0103 Pre-Gummed